# Food & Holiness

### THE DANGERS OF IDOLIZING FOOD

**CHARLENE RALPH**

CLAY BRIDGES
PRESS

**Food & Holiness: The Dangers of Idolizing Food**
Copyright © 2025 by Charlene Ralph

Published by Clay Bridges Press in Houston, TX
www.ClayBridgesPress.com

All rights reserved. No part of this publication may be reproduced, stored in a retrieval system, or transmitted in any form by any means, electronic, mechanical, photocopy, recording, or otherwise, without the prior permission of the publisher, except as provided for by USA copyright law.

Unless otherwise indicated, scripture quotations are taken from the (NASB®) New American Standard Bible®, Copyright © 1960, 1971, 1977, 1995, 2020 by The Lockman Foundation. Used by permission. All rights reserved. www.lockman.org

eISBN: 978-1-68488-131-4
ISBN: 978-1-68488-130-7

Special Sales: Most Clay Bridges titles are available in special quantity discounts. Custom imprinting or excerpting can also be done to fit special needs. Contact Clay Bridges at Info@ClayBridgesPress.com imprinting or excerpting can also be done to fit special needs. Contact Lucid Books at Info@LucidBooks.com.

# Table of Contents

| | | |
|---|---|---|
| Acknowledgments | | v |
| Introduction | | 1 |
| Chapter 1 | Holiness Is the Basis for Happiness | 5 |
| Chapter 2 | Happiness Comes from Obeying God | 18 |
| Chapter 3 | The Duty and Delight of Obeying God | 30 |
| Chapter 4 | We Are Not Our Own | 53 |
| Chapter 5 | We Are God's Stewards | 58 |
| Chapter 6 | Our Bodies and Our Beliefs | 67 |
| Chapter 7 | Our Bodies and Our Effectiveness | 86 |
| Chapter 8 | Our Food and Our Fidelity | 101 |
| Chapter 9 | Food and Our Definition of It | 109 |
| Chapter 10 | Our Goals, Our Weakness, and Our Power | 119 |
| Chapter 11 | How We Function | 143 |
| Chapter 12 | What We Look Like | 152 |
| Chapter 13 | Why We Live | 166 |
| About the Author | | 175 |

# Acknowledgments

Thanks be to God my Father who chose me, my Savior who redeemed me, and the Holy Spirit who dwells within me. I thank God for His daily attendance upon me, to reprove and teach me making me more like Jesus, to lead and guide me making clear His mission for me, and for His provision enabling me to accomplish the purpose He has for me. Though I never even dreamed of writing a book, *Food & Holiness* is just one of the many results of the God-wrought obedience in my life.

Thanks also to Dennis Hobbs, a one-time youth pastor at my church, whom I asked to read through the manuscript of this book, mainly looking for theological accuracy. I am grateful that he took the time even though his family and ministry responsibilities easily took all of his time.

To my twin sister, Cat, only God truly knows how valuable you are to me in this world and what joy it is to contemplate being together for eternity.

# Introduction

*It is not good to eat much honey.*

Food. What is it? Where does it come from? Why do we eat it? These are questions that are not often asked and therefore rarely answered. That is unfortunate and, more importantly, dangerous because the correct answers are absolutely necessary to our well-being. To put it simply, food can be deadly. How can that be, you may ask? After all, we're only talking about food—simple, innocent food. It just sits there waiting to be eaten—harmless, it would seem. In and of itself, food is an inanimate object no more dangerous than, say, a pillow. But when we answer the questions "What is it?" and "Why do we eat it?" the danger becomes very clear. And for those of us who love God and have a heart to want to live for Him, the danger of food is very real.

This book is really not about food but about holiness. God calls us to live holy lives, and for some of us, food is the main culprit in hindering us in our pursuit of holiness. More accurately, it is the way we use food that derails us from living holy lives. We don't eat just to simply give our bodies the nutrition that they need. We also eat for enjoyment. For some of us, the enjoyment aspect overtakes the nutritional aspect and thus creates a problem. We may not recognize that there is a problem, but for most of us, guilt about how and what we eat ought to show us that food is a prominent actor in our spiritual condition. When we eat what we think is too much or isn't good for us, we feel guilty. That is a good thing because just like touching a hot stove, it is the evidence we need to know that our relationship with food is getting in the way of our relationship with God.

I know how that feels because I have lived it. In my case, the way I've used food hasn't simply affected my relationship with God; it was adultery against Him. That word may seem too strong, like one that we think of only in terms of being unfaithful in a marriage, but the key word is *unfaithful*. That's really what adultery is. It's not just loving one thing more than another; it's loving anything else more than the one thing you're supposed to love the most.

I've been a believer in Jesus Christ for as long as I can remember, but I didn't always live like it. I used to love food more than anything. It was my main attraction. I indulged in it without restraint and ate whatever I wanted, whenever I wanted it. Back then, I didn't consider this a problem between me and God. I had separated my life into compartments, putting God in one area and my food god in another. And I never let them cross paths, just like being unfaithful in a marriage. But unlike adultery that the spouse doesn't know about, God knew all about my adultery with food while I continued to deny it. I deceived myself for years and years, never admitting that the way I used food was wrong because subconsciously I knew that would mean I would have to give it all up.

As I gained weight, my appearance also became a big issue to me, and I began to try to lose weight. Trying to limit how much I indulged in my food god was, up to that point in my life, the most painful and difficult thing I had ever tried to do. It went against every desire I had and was at odds with what even made sense to me. Why did I have to push my food god away? How could I possibly limit my enjoyment of my god?

# INTRODUCTION

As you may well know, if you value food as I did, trying to diet to lose weight is a fight you can't win. It's very similar to an adulterous relationship with a person. A person knows that they shouldn't be in it, and they try to say no, and maybe they hold out for a while, but then their heart is drawn back, and they give in. Eventually though, adulterous relationships come to an end in one way or another, but our relationship with food can't completely end like that. Back in the day, I wished it could be, though. I wished there were such a thing as "food pills" that would give me the nutrition I needed so that I could just say "No" to food entirely. Obviously, that was not an option, so I had to learn to live in right relationship with food.

Over time, God began to ask me questions like these: What exactly is it that you don't want to give up? Is it the misery of being overweight and hating it? Is it the slavishness of excess and undisciplined eating that never results in being satisfied? Is it the weariness of trying to fight to control yourself all of the time but always failing? Having come to the end of my rope and having tried everything to overcome the misery, weariness, and lack of discipline, I became willing to answer these questions. In His mercy, God brought me to see the futility of trying to satisfy my soul with food. Eventually, I began to see that eating whatever and however I wanted was not freedom at all but slavery to a god that never gave enough.

By God's grace, I admitted my adultery against Him with my food god, and He changed my heart. I came to accept and to live according to the fact that our hearts and souls are made to indulge in God, to savor Him, to take Him in, to enjoy Him without restraint and without limit. The true God began to be the God I worshiped, and my relationship with food began to change.

The thing I had struggled with the most was sugary foods—cookies, cakes, and ice cream. As my love for God increased, I became able and willing to give all that up. My first step was to stop eating anything with white, refined sugar in it. When I started—and this is more than 30 years ago—I decided that would be for the rest of my life. I kind of did the "food pill" thing and totally stopped eating sugar. I figured that if I couldn't moderate it, I'd just say no altogether. After a year and three months, I had lost 55 pounds and was a whole new person, not only outside but more importantly on the inside.

My relationship with God had grown a lot, and I loved Him more than anything. One day as some family members and I were going out for ice cream (I always went just to be sociable, but I didn't eat it), they were shocked when I said I would have some too. I was also a little shocked, but in that moment, God spoke to me and said that not eating sugar was over. I followed His lead and have had no problems since then with overindulging in sugar.

God remained my only God, and I was in His hands, trusting Him to be all I needed. He had miraculously transformed my relationship with food and caused me to let go of all the sinful ways I had related to food. I gave everything up to Him, all that I thought I couldn't live without, and He enabled me to do all the things I had uselessly struggled to try to do by myself. When God says He is our Savior, He really means it. This whole process, though, was not easy and took decades. It continues to this very day.

As I stated before, this book is not about food but about holiness. Food is just one of the myriad things that we fashion into gods for ourselves. Of these many gods in our lives, one or two are usually the most prominent, and for me that was food. If that is also yours in the fight for holiness, I hope and pray that this book will be a means God will use to set you free from the tyranny of it.

CHAPTER 1

# Holiness Is the Basis for Happiness

*Because it is written, "You shall be holy for I am holy."*

I love heavy, theological books. You know, the ones that are about 5 inches thick and filled with footnotes and references, and when you read them, it's like, *Man, these guys know what they're talking about!* I love them because books like these are all about *God*. That's what the word *theology* means—the study of God.

On the other hand, I really dislike Christian self-help books. You know, the ones that say, "Ten steps to bliss in the Christian life." They are very light on theology or actually get it wrong. Many of them make *people* the focus and not God, which will not help anyone. But sometimes the format is helpful because taking certain steps in a certain order is necessary to accomplish something.

We need deep theology, and we also need direction and help, but they are not mutually exclusive. Good, solid theology is necessary for us to be helped, and enumerating certain steps we need to take is also necessary. Basically, we need a biblically based prescription. So, while this is obviously not a heavy theological book, neither is it one of those Christian self-help books. But I hope and pray that it is an effective and useful combination of both.

## What Good Is Holiness, and Why Should We Seek It?

Some of you may be saying, "Yeah, I'd like to know what good holiness is, because I read the Table of Contents, and Chapter 2 says we're supposed to *sacrifice* for it Or maybe you're wondering what holiness even *is*.

To put it simply, holiness is being perfect, pure, and set apart from all that is imperfect and impure. I'll go into that in detail in a minute, but first let's answer this question: What good is holiness? Holiness has everything to do with happiness. *What?* you may think. *We have to be holy to be happy? That sounds like something monks strive for, living in their monasteries, and from what I've seen, they don't seem all that joyous.* That may well be true, but it remains that holiness is the only way to happiness.

Now, I know this may be coming off sounding all theological and serious, but that's because it is. Holiness is the only way to true happiness because holiness is the only way to God, and God is the ultimate source of happiness. He *knows* what will make us truly happy because He created us, and that is why He commands us to be holy.

Unfortunately, most people are convinced that they know what will work and then spend their whole lives trying it their own way. They try more, better, or different things, only to keep coming up short. They believe that someday they're going to find the satisfaction they seek. But they don't, and they're still working and waiting for the day that they do. I lived like that all my growing up and young adult life, and after all that effort and sacrifice, I still came up empty-handed. Maybe you can see how you've been doing that, and you know what I mean. Hopefully, the rest of this chapter will effectively explain how holiness equals happiness and, by God's grace, take the bones of what I have just said, and put some meat on them. I mean, who doesn't like meaty goodness?

## Commanded to Seek Holiness

At our core, we don't like being commanded to do anything. But God's command to every person is that they be holy. That is theology. That is what is true about God. He commands us to be holy because He wants us to be happy. There's no sugarcoating it or trying not to be dogmatic about it. It just simply *is*. And *how* it is, is simple too, though it may be hard to accept.

It's like when we were growing up; dad told us how it was going to be, whether we liked it or not. If he was a good dad, he had your best interests at heart and did everything he could to make you happy. That doesn't mean he let you skip school and have ice cream for breakfast, which really would make a 10-year-old happy. If that was dad's way, then he would likely buy his 16-year-old a car and let the kid sit at home and play video games. Later on, his now 20-year-old son is still sitting at home, living there for free with no job. You can see that things won't go well for that now adult child. His dad didn't set the rules, certainly didn't discipline him, and didn't require anything from him. Nobody really wants to be raised that way because in the end it makes for a dysfunctional adult who is never happy with anything.

Now, if dad is wise and wants his son to be truly happy, he will require him to eat a good breakfast, go to school, do his chores, get a job, and pay for his own car. There will be a lot of rules, requirements, and sacrifices for the son. But in the end, he has learned the value of hard work and has the ability to rightly enjoy things and likely has a good relationship with his dad too.

So it is with God and us in a certain sense. He lays out the ground rules and requires us to obey them with the intent to make us happy. Now this is where the rub is, just like it was with our own dads as we grew up. We didn't like the rules. At the time, obeying the rules didn't make us happy; it made us mad that we had to do *work*, especially on Saturdays when we were free from school. It just wasn't fair. And we also didn't understand or believe that what dad required was for our good. But we know now that it was. So let us also believe that God intends for our good as well, because He does.

## Father or Just "God"?

Does God intend good for *every* person? To put it simply, no. It depends on our relationship to Him. It's like how, if our dads were good dads, they loved us and took care of us as we grew up, providing all of our needs. Dad made sure we had all we needed, and he did what he needed to do in order to provide for us. He cared about our friends, too, but not in quite the same way because his role for them was not being their dad. Now if there was a tragedy and one of our friends lost his parents and our dad adopted him, then he would be treated and loved the same as us.

It's true that God loves everyone in this world. as is so often quoted in John 3:16, but He doesn't love everyone *the same*. Those who truly call Him their God and Father are loved by Him like He is their dad. But people who don't have a relationship with God are only loved by Him in a general sense. He is not in the role of being their father. They may speak His name, but it is most often done carelessly and sometimes profanely when they say, "Oh my God!" It's a terrible phrase, and I dislike even writing it, but it is what many people say. And they don't even think about what they are actually saying. The all-powerful, all-knowing God of the universe hears them, but do they really mean *my* God? Probably not.

I want to digress a bit to make a really important point: people who use this phrase in a meaningless way have no idea of the peril they are in. Consider the words of Jesus in Matthew 12:36: "But I tell you that every careless word that people speak, they shall give an accounting for it in the day of judgment." Not to get too theological, but the word "*careless*" in this text means to be idle, unfruitful, or useless, like standing around doing nothing. That is the way most people use "Oh my God," to their detriment and the dishonoring of God. Maybe worse than actually saying that is the dumbed-down version, "OMG" that people use in texts. They might say, "Oh, I don't mean anything by it," but that's exactly the point. If we *meant it* when we said it, we would say, "Oh *my* God, my Savior, my Father, the One who loves me and has saved me." Well, look, that is obviously my feeling and belief about that, but the question is, is God really *your* God? Do you *know* Him? There is no more important answer you will ever give in your life than that one.

## Unapproved!

I doubt that anybody likes the word *unapproved*. We don't like being unapproved for a loan or a job. Our parents first taught us the meaning of this word when they disapproved of us, sometimes rightly. But more often than not it felt like it was wrongly. Some of us felt it much worse than others and to this day may still be affected by our parents' disapproval. As I write this, I am 58 years old and still struggle with the shame I felt from being disapproved of. This disapproval we felt from our parents was terrible, and we couldn't do anything about it. The deed was done (or *not* done), and there was no doing it over. We felt shame and took the punishment, but life goes on, and we had to get over it, hoping to do better next time.

But God disapproves of people too. Nobody likes to think of God as being disapproving, but that's the way it is. That's because

He has set certain standards that we are supposed to live up to. Consider the following:

> *As obedient children, do not be conformed to the former lusts which were yours in your ignorance, but like the Holy One who called you, be holy yourselves also in all your behavior; because it is written, "You shall be holy, for I am holy."*
>
> —1 Pet. 1:14–16

Here we are commanded to be obedient children, holy in all our behavior. That is a big ask. Holy in *all* our behavior? And what does *holy* mean anyway? To be holy is to be pure, faultless, sinless, righteous, and set apart—separated from that which is unholy and unclean. Yikes! We are not any of those things.

How can God command us to *be* something that we are not and also to *do* what we cannot do? Surely God's disapproval of us is justified if this is the standard. But let's make it worse and also consider Matthew 5:48: "Therefore you are to be perfect, as your heavenly Father is perfect."

Like, whoa! Who can be *perfect*? That sounds a lot like being holy though, so what's the difference? I'd say that being holy is how we are to *be*, and being perfect (which also means to be holy) has the connotation of constancy, like never *not* being holy. So hopefully you feel bad enough and hopeless enough now to admit that you can't be or do any of this. That would be a good place to be and in agreement with this bit of scripture: "And looking at *them* Jesus said to them, 'With people this is impossible, but with God all things are possible." [Matthew 19:26].

Admitting and knowing deep down that we are flawed and helpless beings is the first step. But consider the previous two passages carefully, and you will see that only those who are the children of God and have Him as their Father are required to be holy and perfect. Whew! you might think, "That lets me off the hook!" And maybe it does, but if you're in that camp where God is not your Father, then you have greater problems than not having to live up to being holy and perfect. But we will get to that later.

Another more important aspect of the word *perfect* means to be complete, to have come to a conclusion, or to have reached the ultimate goal. Well, what does *that* mean? You probably feel complete right now, and in some sense you are. You are a *whole* person—mind, body, and spirit.

The incompleteness comes in if your spirit is not alive. Ephesians 2:4 talks about how we were dead in our sin. That doesn't mean physically dead or else we wouldn't even be alive to know we were dead. It means we are dead spiritually, that we have no spiritual life. That separates us from God because He is a spiritual being, and if we are spiritually dead, we cannot relate to Him or truly know Him. It's like when someone is physically dead, they can't interact with someone who is alive. They can't hear or respond if the living person says something to them. Maybe you have heard the words *born again* that are used to refers to Christians. That term means that they have been born spiritually, that they came to have spiritual life. It says born *again,* meaning that first they were born physically, as we all are, and then at some point in their life, they were born or made alive spiritually.

That may be a lot to take in, or you could be saying to yourself, "Well, who cares about this spiritual life stuff and holiness and perfection? I'm good enough as is!" Most people you know would probably agree with this (except maybe your spouse). But our opinion about ourselves is not the standard that counts. God sets the standard, and as we have seen, that standard is holiness and perfection. So, if you are of a willing heart, maybe you're asking what you have to do to be made holy and therefore be acceptable to God.

## You're Approved!

You gotta love the phrase "you're approved." Who doesn't like to be approved? It's like when you're at the checkout in a store to buy something and you insert your credit card into the credit card thingie, and when the transaction is complete, the screen displays these words, "You're approved!" Don't you feel good when you see that? I do. It's nice to be approved like that, and in a way that's what God has to do for us if we are to become holy and spiritually alive.

First of all, you will be relieved to know that you can't *do* anything to be holy and complete. So, no worries about having to work hard to accomplish that. How does this happen? To put it simply, God gives us His perfect righteousness and takes away all our sin.

If He did that with our credit card, we'd have no debt and a zero balance! That would be nice, but it utterly fails in comparison to the significance of having our whole being—our very lives, our hearts, and souls—approved by God.

So, you may be thinking, *can it be that simple?* It is. As I am writing this—and knowing that God already knows every single person who will read this—my prayer is that you will accept that we are all born sinners, that we do what we know is wrong, and that we are unrighteous and are therefore guilty before God. The amount of our "spiritual debt" that we owe to God because of our sins is higher than we could ever pay. Maybe you have struggled with credit card debt and can't see any light at the end of the tunnel. You're trying to make minimum payments, but the debt only seems to increase.

Have you ever wished you knew a millionaire who would just pay it all off for you? In a sense, Jesus can be that millionaire for your soul. His perfect righteousness is what you need to "pay off" your debt to God. All your sin, guilt, and shame from what you've done and how you've lived can be wiped away. Jesus can be your Savior in all of this. Indeed, He is the *only One* who can since He is the only One who stood in our place to receive the penalty that our sins deserved. He took the debt of all our sins against God upon Himself, as if they were His own, and paid for it by enduring the penalty of an eternal death. In 1 Corinthians 15:3–5, the Apostle Paul wrote:

> *For I delivered to you as of first importance what I also received, that Christ died for our sins according to the Scriptures, and that He was buried, and that He was raised on the third day according to the Scriptures, and that He appeared to Cephas, then to the twelve.*

When Jesus died on the cross, He took your debt upon Himself. He then rose from the dead, now able to forgive your sins. But you must *ask* for the debt to be canceled and removed from you. This takes a serious admission from you that you are indeed guilty of sin, in debt to God, and totally unable to pay.

> *When you were dead in your transgressions and the uncircumcision of your flesh, He made you alive together with Him, having forgiven us all our transgressions, having canceled out the certificate of debt consisting of decrees against us, which was hostile to us; and He has taken it out of the way, having nailed it to the cross.*
> —Col. 2:13–14

Notice the phrase "the certificate of debt consisting of decrees against us." The word *decrees* means God's law, in which He commands us to never lie, cheat, steal, or be envious of what someone else has. And there are many more, but in just these few, we can see that we have broken His law. This is the "certificate of debt" against us because we have failed to perfectly keep God's commands. But as the passage says, Jesus took that debt and canceled it for us. In place of that, He put Himself, having perfectly kept God's commands so that His perfect life can be credited as yours. I hope and pray that if you do not have the spiritual life that comes from accepting Christ as your Savior, you will indeed confess your sins, receive Him, and as the passage says, be made "alive together with Him." If you do so, you will be forgiven by God and accepted as His own. He will adopt you into the family of God and call you a son or daughter. Then He will not only be your God but your Father as well.

## Dude, What's Your Problem?!

So, after all this talk about being holy and perfect and made complete, how come nobody acts that way? Whether we are Christians or not, our behavior is rarely holy, so what gives?! Why do we go on breaking God's law? If He has made us holy and perfect, shouldn't we act like it? Yes, we should, but there is a problem.

Now this has to get theological, but theology doesn't have to be hard to understand and hopefully, by God's grace, I will explain it well. So here goes.

When we are born again, a lot of important things happen. As we've already seen, when we ask to be forgiven and God forgives us, He removes our sin and in place of that gives us the righteousness of Christ. It's kind of like our credit card getting paid off. This is called "imputed righteousness," which means it is given into your spiritual "account."

> *Now to the one who works, his wage is not credited as a favor, but as what is due. But to the one who does not work, but believes in Him who justifies the ungodly, his faith is credited as righteousness.*
> —Rom. 4:4–5

Recall what I said in the previous section—you can't *do* anything to be holy and complete. So, no worries about having to work hard to accomplish that. That is what this Scripture passage means, that

## HOLINESS IS THE BASIS FOR HAPPINESS

you can't *earn* righteousness by what you do, like how you earn a paycheck. You simply have to *believe,* and then righteousness is given to you through your faith in Jesus.

Notice the word *justifies* in that passage. Or actually, let's look at the whole phrase, "Him who justifies the ungodly." That means God declares the guilty person to be innocent. Now, this sounds unjust, like if someone who had committed a mass shooting and killed many people was caught and found guilty, and the judge says, "I declare you innocent." Everyone in that courtroom would gasp and then explode in disagreement, crying out for justice to be done — except, of course, for the murderer. He would feel pretty good about the outcome. But how fair is that? Somebody has to pay! But somebody *did* pay. In this scenario, it's as if the judge's own son stepped up and was put to death in place of the murderer. Jesus stood in our place like that, and we get off scot-free. Indeed, how fair is *that* to Jesus? But that's what He willingly chose to do for us. That's how much He loves us and how much He was willing to pay to save us from what we all deserved.

Whew! That is deep, meaningful stuff, but we must move on. The first point is that the way we are righteous, perfect, and holy is because God *declares* us to be, not because we actually *are*. In theological terms, that is called *justification*. We are justified or "made just." Romans 8:1 puts it like this: "Therefore there is now no condemnation for those who are in Christ Jesus." We are no longer considered guilty and are therefore not condemned. To put it simply, God approves us, and that's all good. It's a done deal, and big changes occur in our hearts and souls. But there is one thing that doesn't change in us, and that is our sin nature. So yes, on the one hand, God has judicially declared us holy and complete, but on the other hand, we are still technically sinners, although forgiven. That leaves us with all the inherent propensities to do what is wrong in order to serve our own selfish desires. The Apostle

Paul, though born again, laments this part of himself when he cries out, "Wretched man that I am! Who will set me free from the body of this death?" (Romans 7:24).

Those are strong words—"body of this death." But we all know this part of ourselves, the part that seems to override what we really want to do. Some of us know this most acutely when we are dieting to lose weight and take that second serving of chocolate cake when we shouldn't have even had the first one. Again, Paul speaks for us when he said, "For what I am doing, I do not understand; for I am not practicing what I *would* like to *do*, but I am doing the very thing I hate" (Romans 7:15).

How true is that? Chocolate cake shouldn't rule over us like that, but sometimes it does. Well, look, we'll get into that later, about how to consistently win the battle with food. But for now, we need to understand the foundation that we stand on in order to succeed. The Bible calls the part of us that causes us to do wrong our "flesh," and there is nothing good about that. Paul puts the blame for his wrongdoing squarely on his flesh, or sin nature.

> *So now, no longer am I the one doing it, but sin which dwells in me. For I know that nothing good dwells in me, that is, in my flesh; for the willing is present in me, but the doing of the good is not.*
>
> —Rom. 7:17–18

This "flesh" part of us is a big problem if we are going to live up to what God has already declared us to be—holy. God commands us not only to *be* holy but also to *act* holy. "But like the Holy One who called you, be holy yourselves also in all *your* behavior; because it is written, 'You shall be holy, for I am holy'" ( Peter 1:15-16). If we have been born again, God has already taken care of the *being* holy part by declaring us to be so, but the *acting* holy is the difficult part.

## We Are Not Alone…

Sounds kind of creepy, like one of those UFO movies where extraterrestrial beings come to Earth and then there are all kinds of problems and someone goes missing and then the army gets involved and there's a scientist who thinks he can explain everything… Anyway, that doesn't have much to do with the point except to say that when we are born again, another thing that happens is that the Holy Spirit of God comes to dwell within us. We are no longer alone. Jesus says in John 14:26, "But the Helper, the Holy Spirit, whom the Father will send in My name, He will teach you all things and bring to your remembrance all that I said to you." Second Corinthians 6:16 says, "For we are the temple of the living God; just as God said, 'I will dwell in them and walk among them; and I will be their God, and they shall be My people.'"

As born-again believers, God dwells in us. The very presence and power of God is the Holy Spirit within us. It is He that will enable us to overcome our sin nature and do the good that we truly want to do. There is much more to say about this, and we will get into that in subsequent chapters, but suffice it to say that God has not left us alone. He is *with us* to empower us to live holy lives.

CHAPTER 2

# Happiness Comes from Obeying God

So, I started Chapter One saying that "Holiness is the only way to true happiness because holiness is the only way to God, and God is the ultimate source of happiness." Then I explained that to be holy, we must be brought to life spiritually, declared holy by God, and then empowered by Him to live holy lives. That is the foundation we need, but it doesn't really explain how it works out practically in our lives. I mean really, how does holiness equal happiness? Maybe I'm a little ahead of myself by saying we need to sacrifice for holiness when I haven't really fleshed out how being holy makes us happy. But by God's grace, hopefully this chapter will do that. Surely, if we are going to sacrifice for holiness, we need to know what we will get for it and that it will be worth it.

## What Is Happiness?

What really *is* happiness? If we're supposed to get happiness by living holy lives, what exactly is it? On the surface, that may seem like a dumb question. I mean, duh, happiness means being happy, right? But being happy in *what* or in *whom*? Happiness doesn't start and end with ourselves. Imagine being in a place that has nothing, like a room that has a white ceiling, white walls, and a white floor, all smooth and featureless. There is nothing to be happy *in* or happy *with*. No person who ever existed could be happy in a place like that.

Even if the room has mirrors, the biggest narcissist in the world who was dashingly handsome or stunningly beautiful with the perfect personality would eventually get bored and dissatisfied with themselves. We need more. We need *stuff* like chocolate cake, a brand-new phone and good friends and a job that pays the bills and reading a good book and sports teams to root for and a vacation in the Bahamas and fun hobbies and the car you've always wanted and a comfortable house and good health and a nice family and the list could go on and on. Having and enjoying all of this is happiness, right?

Now, if you're like some people, you won't want to answer because it sounds like a trick question. And it kind of is, because the answer to it is yes *and* no. Don't you just love that kind of an answer? I don't. I'm a black-and-white kind of person. It's either yes or no, and there can't be two right answers to the same question!

Well, I admit now that there can be two right answers, and in this case there *must* be. On the one hand, enjoying these things *is* happiness because they make some people happy and content. On the other hand, having things like these is *not* happiness because some people are not happy or satisfied with them. If having and enjoying stuff and people were all it took to be happy, then it would work for everyone all of the time, but it doesn't.

So, what's the difference? Well, consider water, for example. It satisfies our body's need for it *every time*. It doesn't work for some and not for others. It works the same for everyone. That's why nobody ever complains that it doesn't. No one ever says, "Gee, that water was good, I guess, but I'm just not happy with it. It didn't satisfy me." So why can't *everyone* be satisfied in the same way with the stuff we have, the things we do, and the relationships we have?

Why isn't just *one* piece of that really moist lemon cake with the sweet crusty glaze on top enough every time? Why do some of us go back for seconds and even thirds? Certainly, our body doesn't need more calories. What are we looking for? Do we just want to enjoy more? Certainly, more is enjoyable, but does more *really* satisfy? It's like that with almost everything. If there were just a little more or just a little better, *then* nirvana! But some of us never quite get there, not with food, or relationships, or things we do, or the stuff we have. We think that someday it will be enough. But even billionaires who have all they could ever want can be miserable and unsatisfied. So, what's the deal?

Let's go back to the water analogy. The reason it wholly satisfies the needs of a person is because it is the *ultimate source* for hydration. In a physical sense, it is an end in itself and needs nothing beyond it to make it effective. When we drink as much as our bodies need, we don't want more; we are satisfied. Water has served its purpose, and we have received what we needed and wanted from it. But when it comes to all the other things I've been talking about, stuff that is supposed to satisfy us, there is a whole other dimension to it.

Look at it this way, if food and relationships, and the stuff we have were meant only to meet our physical needs, we would never eat too much or be in a relationship that wasn't good for us. And actually, we would never do anything that is designed to be enjoyable just for the sake of enjoying it because that wouldn't serve any physical need we have. But there is the whole other aspect of what we feel and what we desire. See, we want more than just to meet our physical needs by eating, drinking, and working to provide shelter and clothing. That's why we cook Brussels sprouts in bacon fat and eat them with bits of bacon (at least I do). If it was purely about nutrition, we should just eat them raw. But we want to enjoy them. And we want to be satisfied because the enjoyment isn't really complete until then.

## Satisfaction Guaranteed!

Who doesn't want to have their satisfaction in a product or service guaranteed? Some businesses even offer a 100 percent guarantee as if satisfaction isn't enough. We all want to know we will be satisfied with something before we spend our time, effort, or money to get it. But some things we just have to take a chance on.

Recently, I tried a new flavor of sparkling water. All the other flavors I had tried in this brand were really good, so I had high hopes for the watermelon flavor. I'll bet you sense the disappointment already. Yeah, I was disappointed because it tasted like cucumber juice! Not good! I don't doubt that the store would return my money, but that's a pain to have to take it back, so I figure just suffer through the rest of it. I just wanted it to be good and it wasn't! Disappointment! Dissatisfaction! We want satisfaction guaranteed!

The misleading thing about this statement is that no one can guarantee that you will be satisfied with something, only that you will get your money back if you aren't. You'll still be unsatisfied. So, what's the point? Well, when we consider that enjoyment isn't complete until we are satisfied, we certainly are going to want to know what it takes to be truly satisfied. And we wouldn't mind a guarantee either.

## What Do You Expect?!

Disappointment and dissatisfaction are the result of expectations that were too high. Well, maybe not too high but misplaced. Generally, if we are disappointed in something, it's because we expected something different than we got. When it comes to the happiness that we get from the things we enjoy, we must have right expectations. I think it is a good rule of thumb to say that if we are disappointed or unsatisfied with something that *ought* to have satisfied us, we expected too much from it. We made too much out of it. In fact, we made it into what the Bible calls an idol.

In this sense, an idol is anything we value more than the thing we ought to value the most. For example, if we are trying to lose some body fat, what we must value most is doing some fasting and getting in some exercise. But if we overindulge in our favorite flavor of ice cream, we have valued that higher than our goal to lose weight and have thus made ice cream an idol. Now, there are myriad things we can idolize, and almost minute by minute we make decisions between two things, choosing which is more important—what we ought to value more and what we ought to value less. It could get confusing, but to put it simply and to set down an absolute, anything that we love and value more than we love and value God is an idol to us.

So how does that relate to happiness? Well, our desire to enjoy things has as its end goal to be satisfied with them, but most things seem to fall short of that. Why? It's because most of us have God in the wrong place in our equation. When we go for the second or third piece of cake, that tells us we were not satisfied with the first piece. In a sense, it failed us and didn't deliver what we wanted. That's because our expectations were wrong. They were in the wrong place. That's why relationships with other people go bad and breakups and divorce are the result. Basically, we expect people and things to provide more for us than they are designed to do. We turn them into idols. We make them a god to us and demand that they deliver what we want.

We can see vividly how this works in relationships between people. Imagine that a man falls in love with a woman, and she responds in kind. They are crazy about each other and declare their undying love, feeling happier than they ever thought possible. But you know how it goes. Pretty soon, the guy is finding stuff he doesn't like about the woman, or she begins to dislike stuff about the guy. They disagree on things, and then friction, anger, division, and perhaps followed by unfaithfulness. So what gives? To put it frankly, they were just using each other. All of the warm, fuzzy love they felt for each other was wholly dependent on them getting what they wanted from the other. When the other person was no longer what satisfied them, the "love" was over and in many cases turned to hate.

This is the grizzly result when one person turns another person into an idol, when they exalt them as their god and want them to satisfy all their expectations and desires. When the other person fails to live up to "God" status, the relationship ends, and the person is literally discarded as worthless. In a situation like that, no human being can ever live up to what the other person wants. Love that does not *always* love isn't really love at all.

In a similar way, we tend to use the things we have or the things we do to satisfy our needs and desires. They become idols or gods to us, and we demand that they satisfy us. When they don't, we try harder, indulge more, or spend more trying to squeeze out of them what we want. It's futility.

## The Great Beyond

For more people than not, there is this vague and undefined "beyond" that their hearts long for, when things will finally be "enough." What most don't want to admit, though, is that this "beyond" is actually God Himself. People unknowingly seek Him, but in all the wrong places and in all the wrong ways. It's kind of like when we get hungry and then *really* hungry, there is this gnawing inside that must be satisfied. It doesn't let up, and makes us irritable and distracted, and nearly unable to enjoy anything at all.

There is a spiritual place inside us like that. We try to fill it with things and experiences, but only God Himself can fill the spiritual hunger that is in us. We must have our hearts and souls fed and satisfied by Him. *God* must be our God, the One we must value more than anything or anyone else. When that is the case, we are in a place to rightly and freely enjoy the things of this life. When we get this equation right, everything works—no more fighting with ourselves to say no to more dessert, no more trying harder to lose weight, no more forcing ourselves to shut off the football game and go read our Bible. Well, it's not really that easy and doesn't happen that suddenly, but as we get more and more in line with God, eventually it will.

## There's Only One Way

It seems kind of narrow to say that there is only one way, that to be happy and content, we have to do it God's way. But it's like that with more things than you might think. First and foremost, it is how a person gets right with God.

There are not "many ways to God" as some assert. There is only one way—repent of your sin, humbly and sincerely ask God to forgive you, and He will remove the guilt of your sin and give you the righteousness of Christ. Any other way that people say takes you to God doesn't have provisions for how your sin is removed.

Or take being hungry. There is only one way to not be hungry—eat! Or maybe your lawn is a bit long and needs mowing. How many ways are there to make the grass shorter? As we know, there is only one way—cut it! So, we should not be surprised or object that there is only one way to be truly happy in this world.

## How Holiness Equals Happiness

In the first chapter, we saw what it means for God to be our God—that we must be born again, to go from being spiritually dead to spiritually alive, with the Holy Spirit dwelling in us so that we are in a right and living relationship with God. We have also seen that much of the time; we don't act like He is our God because we value other things more than Him.

This is the point where we must turn from talking about happiness to talking about holiness. Why? Because seeking to live a holy life is the only way to have God in the right place in our hearts, with the consequence that everything else in our lives will fall into line behind that.

People who live holy lives seek God first. He is their primary focus and the One to whom they have wholly submitted themselves. They consider themselves His servants, to do His will and to accomplish His purposes. They depend on Him for strength and trust Him to provide for them. God is their highest and chief joy in life, their ultimate happiness. They find that their hearts and souls are satisfied in Him alone. They love Him more than anything, and as a result, they love other people and seek to communicate God's love to them in all they do.

And because God is truly their God, they don't struggle with overindulging in anything. Wait a minute! For real? No more struggle? Well, no, not really. There will still be a struggle. But when God is our God, our propensity to overdo things will be greatly lessened, because we no longer consider the stuff we have or the things we do as our ultimate source of happiness and satisfaction. *God* is that for us. I mean, that really is the key point of this whole book. If you really get that, you wouldn't have to even read any more, but the rest of this book will help you see how that all works out.

So yeah, the struggle is there, but those who seek to live holy lives focus their fight on being holy, not on trying to be moderate with the things of this world. Holiness takes care of that.

## Is it Really All About Happiness?

No, it is not all about happiness, not by a long shot. But God *does* command us to be happy. Consider these commands to be happy in God:

*Delight yourself in the Lord.*

—Ps. 37:4

*And you shall rejoice before the L<small>ORD</small> your God.*
—Deut. 16:11

*Rejoice in the Lord always; again I will say, rejoice!*
—Phil. 4:4

These are commands to be happy in God.

Now, this could lead to a whole long discussion on what this means exactly, like how can you be *commanded* to be happy? Isn't happiness just a spontaneous feeling? Yes, it is. But it is more than that and something we will get into later. Really that subject could be a whole book in itself, and there is one out there that I highly recommend—*Desiring God* by John Piper. The book fleshes out its main point: "The chief end of man is to glorify God by enjoying Him forever." It makes the point better than any other book except the Bible, so maybe you want to read that and then come back and finish this book.

Of course, if you read that book and apply what's in it, you wouldn't need this one anymore. But if you want to keep reading this one, here it is. Let's just say that God *commands us* to delight and rejoice in Him because He wants us to be happy and that living a holy life is necessary to delight in God. So, try this out: imagine you are some kind of robot walking around all stiff and jerky and saying in a monotone voice, "I will oh-bay." Is that what it means to obey God's commandments? In a sense, yes. We are duty-bound to obey God. He requires it like a master requires a slave to do as he says. God doesn't cut us any slack. It's His way or else!

You may think, "Whoa! That doesn't sound very nice!" On the surface, it doesn't. But it's kind of the same as when mom made us eat our broccoli (I say "us" because I have a twin sister). She'd say, "You can sit at the table all night if you want, but you're not getting up until the broccoli is gone!" It was her way or the highway, and to us, it was harsh and unfair. We would try waiting it out, like maybe mom would eventually let us go, but dessert beckoned. Finally, we choked down the broccoli, not only to get dessert but because our favorite evening TV show was about to come on.

As an aside, one time my sister didn't want to finish her hamburger, so when no one was noticing, she stuck it in the butter dish—you know, the rectangular one with the lid. When it was discovered the next day, neither of us would say who did it, and mom, not always being the disciplinarian she should have been, let us get away with it. The funny thing is, though, that to this day, my sister and I can't agree on who actually did the deed. It's like that with lots of things from our growing up. I'll say, "No, I did that," and she'll say, "No, that was me!" and we can't remember well enough to know for sure. Well, anyway, that's off the point, so let's get back to it.

God *does* require obedience like our mom did, and for the same reason, because it is for our good and will, in the end, make us happy.

## We Obey God Because We Love Him

I love to serve my husband. Considering our very difficult and painful 35-year history, this is a miracle, but God has enabled me to truly love to obey my husband. Now, it has been kind of easy, though, because he is really passive and usually doesn't ask me to do anything, but I finally got him to ask for things. Like when he wants something to eat, all he does is open his mouth and point into it. He used to wait to ask until he saw that I was done with whatever I was doing, but I got him trained to command me to serve him immediately. The point is, he commands, and I obey. But I *love* to. That's because I love him and want to please him.

That's how we ought to obey God—not out of duty, though it *is* our duty, but out of delight because we want to please Him. Jesus says in John 14:15, "If you love Me, you will keep My commandments." *Love* is the motivation to obey.

Consider the following:

*If you keep My commandments, you will abide in My love; just as I have kept My Father's commandments and abide in His love. These things I have spoken to you so that My joy may be in you, and that your joy may be made full.*
—John 15:10–11

Here we see that if we obey God, we will abide in His love. To abide means to stay in a place, to be with someone. I can't think of a better place to be than with God Himself, wrapped up in His love. That's where our hearts and souls long to be. We were *made* for that.

Think of your favorite person in the whole world. Don't you just love to be with them? And you can be happy and content with them just being with them. You don't necessarily need some kind of activity. You can just sit and share a cup of coffee. You're *with* them, and it's good. It's enough.

That's how it is between us and God when we abide in His love. He is with us, and we are with Him. Remember the section called "The Great Beyond" some pages ago? I said, "There is a spiritual place inside us. . . . We try to fill it with things and experiences, but only God Himself can fill the spiritual hunger that is in us." That is the very place that gets filled when we abide in God's love, and He abides in us. But as we saw in John 15:10–11, we must keep God's commandments. Okay then, you may ask, what are they?

*The foremost is, "Hear, O Israel! The Lord our God is one Lord; and you shall love the Lord your God with all your heart, and with all your soul, and with all your mind, and with all your strength." The second is this, "You shall love your neighbor as yourself." There is no other commandment greater than these.*
—Mark 12:29–31

Simply put, we must love God and love people. Some may think of God's commandments as the Ten Commandments—all those "Thou shalt nots"—and while it is true that we must obey those, His foremost command that we must love Him, and love people takes care of all the other commandments.

## By-Products

When I think of by-products, I think of stuff that is kind of just free, like you get it for nothing as a result of doing something else. Take sawdust, for example. When you mill wood to get lumber, the by-product is sawdust. No one cuts wood to get sawdust and then throws the lumber away, but when we cut wood for some project, we sweep up the sawdust and throw it out. Lumber mills, though, collect their sawdust and use it in particleboard or sell it as mulch or bedding for small animals. The point is the sawdust is like free money; it's there as a result of doing the main thing—cutting wood. So it is with being truly happy and content. We must do the main thing—pursue holiness—which puts God in the right place in us so we can rightly enjoy and be satisfied with the things we do and the stuff we have. If we try being happy any other way, it's like expecting to get sawdust before you cut the wood.

CHAPTER 3

# The Duty and Delight of Obeying God

If we are convinced that we ought to live holy lives, how practically do we do that? Obviously, keeping God's commandments is the foundation. We must oh-bay! But there are many factors that can keep us from doing that, like feeling that it isn't worth it, or it's too difficult, or we want to do this rather than that. Choosing holiness can be very difficult, but understanding what makes it difficult can make it much easier to choose it. So now it's time for a little math!

**A Math Lesson...**
I'm not good at math at all, not even simple computations. Being very artistically minded, all I wanted to do in high school math class was draw and doodle on my folders. My bent to do that was higher in classes I disliked more than others, and math ranked the highest. Maybe I'd be better at math today if I had learned more about it, but there's no going back now. Calculators weren't invented for nothing, you know.

One thing I heard in math class was the phrase "greater than" or "lesser than," accompanied by some strange symbol. When the teacher used those phrases, it always sounded like only part of a sentence, and in my mind, I said, *Well, greater than what?* And it did not help when the teacher brought the alphabet into it, like "a" is greater than "b." I mean, what the heck? I thought I was in *math* class, you know, like *numbers*? Letters are for English class (also a basic fail for me). About the only thing I got from all that was that one thing can be a larger quantity than another. But I already knew that. And when math class started involving symbols that looked like goofy macaroni, I really checked out.

So, while I am not good at math, I get the basic concept of "greater than" and "lesser than," especially when it comes to what we value in our lives. That is the real key to why choosing to obey God can be so difficult. We have God on the wrong side of the "greater than" symbol.

## It's Not Rocket Science

When it comes to numbers, we know that 4>2, that 2=2, and that 3<6. (I looked that up which way the little thingies had to be pointing, but not the 2=2.) Obviously, numbers are quantities, and no one can dispute that some are greater or lesser than others.

If only it were that simple for us to determine what we value most. If we could just put a number on it! But you know, sometimes we can, like when the newest smartphone becomes available, we may gladly spend $800 to buy it. But would we forego the new phone and give the $800 to our church to give to some missionaries in need of a generator to replace the one that got destroyed in a hurricane? Our answer to that definitely tells us what we value more. But there are many more things that aren't so clear-cut. It's not simple math like that.

Our hearts and minds can fool us almost every time because it is inherent in us to be selfish and seek to satisfy our sinful desires at the cost of nearly everything else. It's actually kind of disturbing how easily we can deceive ourselves into thinking God is number one to us when He isn't. We *must* be able to identify the things we value more than we value God, or we will fail to effectively live holy lives.

Though it can be difficult to identify what our motives are, I think generally we can know what we value the most by what we spend our time and attention on. For instance, I am an artist, and I love to draw, I mean *love* to draw! Many years ago, I was working on a drawing for quite a while in the evening, and then I heard a strange chirping sound. *Hmm, what is that?* I thought. But the sound came from more than one place. And then I looked out my window and saw the sky. It looked like there was light in it. *Strange*, I thought. And then I looked at my clock. It was 5:30 a.m. *It's morning! What I heard were the birds waking up.* I couldn't believe that I was so wrapped up in doing the drawing that I had been at it all night. It seemed like no time at all!

Of course, that was way back when I used to still be up at 1:00 or 2:00 a.m., so it was only another few hours later than that. Now I get up at 6:00 a.m., something about getting older maybe. Anyway, the point is that when we love something, we give our undivided attention to it and are willing to spend all our resources on it. We make decisions all the time about what we love and what we value more than something else. When we choose to eat an orange rather than a cupcake, we show that we value the orange more and most likely value our health more than the yummy goodness of a cupcake. Or we choose to go out into 5-degree Fahrenheit weather with blowing snow to shovel our elderly neighbor's driveway because we value helping them more than our own comfort. Every moment, we're doing math! Always asking ourselves, "Do I consider this to be greater than that?" They can be momentous choices, like choosing to quit your job, sell your house and go to Africa to be a missionary, or as mundane as whether to have white or wheat bread for your toast.

We must be diligent to constantly assess where our heart is, what our motives are, and what we really value the most at any given moment. Do we want to watch TV or read our Bible? I think most of us would only have one answer to that, but do we really live according to it? We have got to choose God in every choice we make. We need to do what best serves His purpose for each of us, from what we eat; how we exercise; what we wear; what we look like; how often we read, study, and memorize the Bible; how much we pray; how much TV we watch; how we respond to people; and on and on. The more we value God in all of these things, the more holy our lives will be. We have got to believe that He is "greater than" all else because He is at the root of every choice we make.

## Where's the Love, Man?

Another aspect to the choices we make is not only do they show whether we value God above all, but do they also show whether we are *obeying* Him or not? Now, these two aspects are kind of the same thing. When our choice is based on valuing God more than anything, it will also be the choice that obeys His will and, in effect, keeps His commandments. But there is a key factor in how and why we will choose God and obey Him, and it's *love*, man!

So, my sister, Cat, and I are avid scale model hobbyists. We put together plastic model kits of 1/24 scale cars and trucks and 1/35 scale military vehicles. We spend weekends at her house in a nice little nook in her basement at a card table arrayed with all kinds of tools, paint, and glue. We love it, but sometimes what we are building can be difficult, and often my sister, in frustration, will say, "Where's the love?!" And if we have just finished a yummy lunch, I will usually say, "We ate it," and she will answer, "Oh yeah."

But frustration with the stuff Cat and I make can be high because we are usually creating our own models out of two or three different kits and using bits and pieces from our "boneyard"—boxes and boxes of stuff from leftover model kits. I wish you could see some of the things we have made! We've made many "rat rods"—a real thing in the custom car culture—but it is a tedious process as we fabricate parts and pieces and try to get our cars (or trucks) to look the way we want them to. It can take six or eight months or more to build one car. It may sound like a lot of tedious, laborious, painstaking, arduous, difficult, exasperating, aggravating—oh sorry, I went on a little bit there! But really it can be like that. But to us, it is worth it because we love the process, and we love the final result even more. The frustration and effort pales in comparison to how much we love to make models. It's all about the love, man! And that's exactly what we need in order to consistently do what God has for us to do.

But we can't just simply keep God's commandments no matter how we feel or what our motives are and then "be holy." We have to *love* to obey Him. For example, say I have some neighbors who are in financial difficulty and living on canned beans. I cook them a nice meal and bring it over. They open the door, and I say, "Here is a dinner for you." They receive it gladly and begin to thank me profusely. But I hold up my hand and say, "No, it's my duty. I could have done a lot of other things than cook that blasted meal, but I'm supposed to love my neighbor, so there it is!" and then I walk away. No one would say that is loving your neighbor, and yet I actually did the loving thing, which was providing a meal.

It's not *what* you do so much as *why* and *how* you do it. For instance, you could rush over to your neighbor's house, smash in the front door, run in, see them taking a nap on the couch, grab them, and drag them out of their house and across the front lawn to the road. Would that be a loving thing to do? Not if the birds are singing, the sun is shining, and it's a wonderful day in the neighborhood. But if their house was on fire, it certainly would be the loving thing to do.

So true holiness depends on the heart, that when we obey God's command to love our neighbor, we do it out of love. This love we need comes from God, but we have to be in right relationship with Him, which means valuing or loving Him more than anything else. He has to be the One who is "greater than" in our lives. When we consider Him so, He pours His love into us, which is the love we need to love our neighbor without "loving" them hypocritically.

Now, if you're really paying attention, you will have noticed a thing about this that doesn't seem to make sense. The love we need to truly love to obey God comes *from* Him. You can only truly love God with the love that *He* gives you, but He only gives you this love if you love Him. It sounds like circular reasoning—you are loved by God only if you love Him, but you can't love Him without getting the love He gives you when you love Him. Whew! Where is a theologian when you need one? In the absence of one, let's just let God Himself tell us through His word.

*We love, because He first loved us.*
—1 John 4:19

So that's simple. This verse goes back to what it means to be redeemed from our sin and given spiritual life: God *loved* us first by dying for us, as the following verse describes:

*But God demonstrates His own love toward us, in that while we were yet sinners, Christ died for us.*
—Rom. 5:8

God started the whole process when He loved us by bringing us into a right relationship with Himself. It's like the chicken and the egg thing. God created the chicken, and then it lays eggs. Simple. So He created us (being born again), and then we love Him and consequently receive His love. As we have seen, holy behavior is not just *doing* the right thing but *loving* to do it—and loving to do it requires receiving the love we need from God.

## The Lumberjack

When you see trees lying on the ground next to stumps and sawdust everywhere, you don't need Sherlock Holmes to tell you that a lumberjack has been there. You can also deduce that the lumberjack had a saw and cut down the trees.

In a previous section, I likened cutting wood to living a holy life and the resulting happiness of a holy life was like sawdust, the by-product. Of course, cutting wood requires some sort of saw and a lumberjack to wield it. The saw in this analogy is what may be termed the "spiritual disciplines" of Bible reading, scripture memorization, studying the Bible, praying, and meditating on scripture. This is not an exhaustive list, but it covers the basics. These are tools, like the saw, and are the means and basic foundation by which we live holy lives. We've got to pick them up and use them as they are intended by God to be used.

Engaging in these disciplines takes effort, like when we try to memorize, it can feel like trying to cut wood by hand with a really dull saw. But simply reading the Bible is easier, like how a chainsaw goes through wood like butter. We'll get into the specifics of these disciplines later, but for now, take heart! The more we engage in these things, the easier it gets! That's part of why they are called "disciplines"—the more you practice them, the more disciplined you get.

## Pursuing and Practicing

Cats are fun to watch, as evidenced by so many cat videos online of cats and kittens doing things. You could literally waste hours and hours going from one video to the next (whoa, did you feel a twinge of conscience there?). Anyway, cats can be very entertaining, and maybe you have one or two. They love to chase things. They stalk them like a wild tiger, eyes as big as saucers, wholly focused on their prey. They will not be distracted but go after it like their life depends on it. They *will* get the thing!

So, we need to be singularly focused on pursuing holiness. We must get it! Now, what do I mean by pursuing holiness? Is it like we have to catch it? Well, sort of. It's like pursuing excellence in playing the piano. It's a goal, a place you're trying to get to, a condition you're trying to reach. Maybe you took piano lessons as a child, really admired your teacher, and wanted to be like them. You practiced all the lessons they gave you, and eventually you began to be able to play like your teacher. In a similar way, we must "practice" the spiritual disciplines so that we become more and more like our teacher—Jesus.

> *A disciple is not above his teacher, nor a slave above his master. It is enough for the disciple that he become like his teacher, and the slave like his master.*
> —Matthew 10:24–25

We must pursue holiness by engaging in the spiritual disciplines, but again I must say, it's not that simple. It's not like we just do those things, and voila! we're like Jesus, holy and perfect. As I have been emphasizing, our hearts must be right with God, and we must do all out of love for Him.

## Sitting under the Son

Not only do we have to depend on God's love to obey Him, but we need His power to obey Him. God's love is the "why," and His power is the "how." Thankfully, His love and power kind of come together. If we're filled with His love, His power is there too. And we *need* it, we can't do anything without it. It would be like trying to cut wood with a chainsaw that isn't turned on. Imagine trying to use it like a hand saw. It would just get snagged on the wood and all hung up and you don't get anywhere. I mean, I tried it once. It's not that the chainsaw doesn't have sharp teeth on it like a handsaw, they are probably sharper, but it isn't made to operate like a handsaw. The chainsaw has its own power and has to be used accordingly to function correctly.

In the same way, we must pick up and engage in the spiritual disciplines as we depend on God's power to make our engagement in them effective. Our progress in holiness depends on that, but what we do is only part of the equation—and an infinitesimally small part at that. Paul describes this in 1 Corinthians 15:10: "But I labored even more than all of them, yet not I, but the grace of God with me." Here, Paul is saying that he worked harder than Peter and the rest of the apostles to proclaim the gospel. But then he takes all of the credit off of himself and credits it to God when he says, "but the grace of God with me." Now the word *grace* may not sound like a word for *power* as it would have to be in this context to make sense, but it is. Jesus uses it in a similar way.

And He [Jesus] has said to me, *"My grace is sufficient for you, for power is perfected in weakness." Most gladly, therefore, I will rather boast about my weaknesses, so that the power of Christ may dwell in me.*

—2 Corinthians. 12:9

Here, the words *power* and *grace* are used synonymously and show that God's grace is expressed as His power. So, the way Paul labored was according to God's power at work in him. But Paul's contribution to his efforts was the infinitesimal, microscopic part. He walked and talked and preached the gospel, but *God*—that's the huge part—was the One who accomplished what Paul did. Whenever we compare anything to God, He is infinitely larger, so when we say we worked to do something, it was God's power that accomplished it in us and for us.

*For it is God who is at work in you, both to will and to work for* His *good pleasure.*

—Philippians 2:13

Lord, *You will establish peace for us, since You have*

*also performed for us all our works.*
—Isaiah 26:12

*Now the God of peace . . . equip you in every good thing to do His will, working in us that which is pleasing in His sight, through Jesus Christ, to whom be the glory forever and ever. Amen.*
—Hebrews 13:20–21

Really, becoming more and more holy in our actions and our character is completely out of our hands. Jesus says:

*I am the vine, you are the branches; he who abides in Me and I in him, he bears much fruit, for apart from Me you can do nothing.*
—John 15:5

Imagine a bunch of grapes talking to each other. "Hey, I was the first one to bud this year!" "Well, *my* blossom was the prettiest!" "Who cares about your blossom!" says another, "*I'm* the biggest grape!" "Well, I'm shinier. I don't have that dull white stuff on *me*!" Ridiculous, right? These grapes didn't do one thing to be what they are!

It's God who causes the growth, and if He doesn't do it, it doesn't happen. He also empowers and manages the whole process of holiness, from putting in us the desire to be holy, moving us to take the actions to be holy, and then creating that holiness within us. There is absolutely nothing we can do to make ourselves holy any more than we can make ourselves warm by sitting in the hot, summer sun. I mean, we *get* warm because we sat in the heat of the sun, but we didn't *do* anything to our bodies to make them warmer. They just got that way from the effects of the sun. So it is with holiness. We become holy by the Holy Spirit causing it to be, but we must engage in the means God uses to make us more and more holy.

## Disciplinary Action Must Be Taken!

Children need to be disciplined, to be taught the difference between right and wrong. They need to learn what is appropriate and what isn't. They need to get *schooled*! In a similar way, when we are born again, we become a new creation in Christ. We're like children and need to learn how to properly operate in our new life. Regardless of how long we have been a believer, we still need teaching and training. That's because we don't remember things very long, and we default back to sin and self-focus. The lessons can be hard and uncomfortable and feel like we're getting ground into powder.

> *Though you pound a fool in a mortar with a pestle along with crushed grain, yet his foolishness will not depart from him.*
>
> —Proverbs. 27:22

Thankfully, we are not technically fools, and God does work to remove our foolish beliefs and correct our foolish actions, but usually it's learning things over and over and over again. Kind of like when mom said, "Don't you ever learn?" Well, we do eventually because God *will* get the job done in us.

God put me through and brought me through a lot. I started a ketogenic way of eating (July 2019), but being basically uninformed about what it took to do it successfully and thinking it was simple and easy, I almost wound up in the hospital. It all had to do with electrolyte balance and the fact that I lost too much weight too fast. I didn't start this way of eating to lose weight but because it is the most effective way to keep blood sugar stable and even. So, I got into a bad spot physically and was as weak as a bunny. My hormones and emotions were all out of whack, and for weeks and weeks I could do nothing but sit around and watch TV. Even walking to the end of my driveway and back was an effort. But God was mightily at work, teaching me that no matter what my emotional, spiritual, and physical conditions are, He is enough for me. That *He has me in His hands and that everything is exactly how it has to be for Him to accomplish His perfect purpose in me for my greatest good.*

Sounds kind of like one of those old church creeds, doesn't it? It did become a creed for me and continues to this day. Apparently, there is no end to me needing to be reminded that this is true as God continues to bring situations and conditions upon me that constantly remind me of this basic truth. It's kind of like military training—having the truth beaten into me so to speak, over and over and over until it finally sticks, and we can get on to the next lesson. At the same time, I never lose my need to remember the basics and then live accordingly. Similarly, we need to be constantly reminded about what is true about God and ourselves and this world. That's where God's word comes in.

## The Whole Truth and Nothing But the Truth

We need the truth. If we try to live our lives based on what is not true, we're doomed to failure—failure in everything. Without truth, we will fail to love God, we will fail to obey Him, we will fail to grow in holiness, and we will fail to love people. I'd say that's a total fail.

Now, there is truth everywhere, like in science books, which contain the truth about our DNA and how our brains work, or books on how to grow tomatoes, or how scales, chords, and notes relate to each other in music, and the list could go on. But the truth we can't live successfully without what is in the Bible. And the ultimate truth that the Bible teaches is this: the chief end of man is to glorify God by enjoying Him forever.

Let's break this down a little bit. "The chief end of man" speaks of our ultimate goal, the thing we strive for as the end point, like a marathon runner reaching the finish line. To "glorify God" is to esteem Him as the most magnificent being in all creation, to treasure

Him, and to value Him above everything and everyone in our lives. "Enjoying Him forever" means just what it says—to enjoy God and be happy in Him, but how it fits with "to glorify God" is that we believe and proclaim how perfectly good and satisfying He is. We need nothing beyond Him. He is our ultimate source for all we need and desire. To proclaim this is to glorify God, and then to live accordingly is to enjoy Him. The "enjoying" part is key, because we don't glorify Him if we aren't enjoying Him. It's like, well, I guess I could get all theological and go into a long explanation but suffice it to say that we must value God above all and seek for all our satisfaction and joy in Him.

This is the truth as found in the Bible, and the whole meaning of our existence. If we believe that this is not true, we will believe something that is false. And if we live according to that false belief, we will suffer unwanted and painful consequences. That's why it is imperative that we read and *know* God's word and then live accordingly. But what exactly *is* God's word, and how does it function in our lives?

## The Living Word

One aspect of God's word is that it is merely ink on paper. The ink is formed to make letters, and letters grouped into words, and words into sentences, and so on until we have a whole book. But it's just paper and ink, like any other book, so what makes it different? Simply put, the Bible is unique among every other book, not only because of its basic content but also because of what it says about itself.

> *All Scripture is inspired by God and profitable for teaching, for reproof, for correction, for training in righteousness.*
>
> —2 Timothy 3:16

> *For the word of God is living and active and sharper than any two-edged sword and piercing as far as the division of soul and spirit, of both joints and marrow, and able to judge the thoughts and intentions of the heart.*
>
> —Heb. 4:12

No other book in the world proves itself to have been written by God Himself (through the agency of man), nor does any other book, religious or otherwise, proclaim that it is alive and prove itself to be so. God's word is living and active in the sense that it is a manifestation of God. It is *alive* and interacts with our spiritual life. It is *active* and accomplishes God's purposes in each one of us. Being alive and active means there is power in it—power to do all kinds of good stuff to us, in us, and through us.

It is also sharper than a sword, cutting right down to the bone, reaching the deepest parts of us, and showing us what is really there. It reveals everything about us and exposes our heart, our motives, and our sin. And we *need* this because we are unable to correctly judge and assess ourselves. We need to know our sin if we are to successfully fight against it. We also need to know God more if our love for Him is to grow and be strong. We need our eyes opened, and that is what the Word of God does. The power, effectiveness, and glory of God's word ought to cause us to say, along with the psalmist, "My heart stands in awe of Your words" (Ps. 119:161).

## When We Value God's Word, We Obey It

However we consider and relate to God's word, whatever our experience of it is, we have to get to the place of *loving* it. We *must* be able to say with Job:

> *I have treasured the words of His mouth more than my necessary food.*
>
> —Job 23:12

When Job said that he treasured God's words, he was finishing this statement:

> *My foot has held fast to His path; I have kept His way and not turned aside. I have not departed from the command of His lips.*
>
> —Job 23:11–12

Job *treasured* God's words and thereby obeyed them. This is similar to Psalm 119:11: "Your word I have treasured in my heart, that I may not sin against You."

The word *treasured* means just what it sounds like—to hold, to keep, and to hide. We naturally do these things with the stuff we love. This all comes together in John 1:11 where Jesus is called the Word, and then in John 14:15 He says, "If you love Me, you will keep My commandments." So, we must love and treasure God's word, not only His written word but also Jesus the Word, with the result that we obey Him!

## Breathing It In

I mentioned before that I eat ketogenically, which means my carbohydrate intake is very low. This excludes many of the foods I used to eat and really enjoyed, like donuts, ice cream, cake, candy bars, and oh! raspberry Zingers! If you know what those are and like them, you know what I mean. Well, I haven't had a crumb of anything like these foods since I changed how I eat and likely never will. For me, the negative impact of refined sugar on my physical being isn't worth the positive impact it can have on my emotional being. Anyway, my husband had a package of fresh baked Danishes and was near me when he opened the package. Man alive! The aroma of those things wafted into my senses and almost knocked me over! I wanted to eat one! Enjoying the aroma just wasn't enough. Well, it had to be because I would no longer eat stuff like that, but it made me think of scripture. How much do we take it in? Can we say with Jeremiah:

*Your words were found and I ate them, and Your words became for me a joy and the delight of my heart; for I have been called by Your name, O Lord God of hosts.*
—Jeremiah 15:16

Merely breathing in the aroma of food does nothing for the needs of our body, but eating *feeds* us. When we take in God's word, how do we do it? Do we "eat" it eagerly and with much enjoyment, or do we just skim over it and just sort of enjoy the aroma? Or is it worse t, that it doesn't even smell that good to us? Unfortunately for most of us, I think we more often sound like this: "You also say, 'My, how tiresome it is!' And you disdainfully sniff at it" (Malachi 1:13). The context of this verse is that God was judging the Jewish priests in the temple for being irreverent in performing the sacrifices. They "did their duty," but they didn't really want to; they had no heart for it. We, too, can be like that when it comes to taking in God's word, but woe to us if we are! We *need* to be in awe of God's word because it is our lifeblood. We can't live without it. To be more specific, we can't live *how God commands us to live* without it.

## Discipline

Ughh! Discipline?! That doesn't sound like any fun! Well, neither is studying for a test, but you do it because you really want to pass it. I can't remember ever studying for a test in middle school or high school, not that I was that smart, but probably because I didn't care that much about passing it. Plus studying means disciplining yourself or your parents making you do it, neither of which happened for me. So, I barely graduated from high school and certainly didn't go on to a college of any sort.

But for those of you who aspired to higher learning for the sake of becoming a doctor, engineer, police officer, chef, psychologist, or any other thing that takes more than a high school degree, you disciplined yourself to learn the stuff you needed to know. Whether you liked it or not, you studied, memorized, thought about, talked about, and focused on the stuff you needed to learn to get the degree you wanted. You *lived* in it. No doubt before a big test, it could well have been said of you, "Yeah, that Steve, he eats, sleeps, and breathes all that biology stuff."

How much more important is it for us as believers? We must wholly depend on God and His word and be similarly committed to studying scripture and *knowing* it. We may not think of it, but spiritually speaking, we are always at some stage of "studying for a test." It's what we know and how much we believe it that will determine how well we respond to testing and difficulties.

## The Basic Four

Probably this idea isn't original with me, that there are basically four modes or ways of taking in God's word, but it's what is occurring to me now, so we'll go with it. We can take in God's word by simply reading it, studying it, memorizing it, and meditating on it. There are lots of different resources for how to go about it, and you likely are already doing those things to some extent, so I'll just outline the basics and also tell you what I do.

One thing I want to emphasize is that these four modes each have a specific and different effect in us, so consistently engaging in all four will give a more well-rounded intake of God's word. Another thing is that to receive the greatest benefit from God's word, we must come to it with clean hands and a pure heart, at least as clean and pure as we can be at the time. When I come to God's word, I get down on my knees and ask God to forgive me of sin, to make me holy, and to make me as pure as possible so I can receive His word as purely and uncorrupted as possible. I thought of literally washing my hands before picking my Bible, but I never started that....

*Reading*

So, this may be the easiest way to get God's word into us — simply reading it. Maybe you have heard of the book *Living by the Book*, written by Howard Hendricks. I highly recommend it. It is a how-to-study-the-Bible book, but it also contains 10 strategies for effective reading. I don't doubt you would benefit from those, plus this book would be mighty helpful when it comes to studying as well.

What I do is read the Bible in the morning and evening, and in so doing, take in parts of the whole Bible every day. In the morning, I read through a couple chapters in the Psalms, one chapter in Proverbs, and a couple chapters in the Gospels. In the evening, I read a couple chapters in the section from Genesis to Job, a couple from Ecclesiastes to Malachi, and a couple in the New Testament, from Acts to Revelation. Eventually, I have read the whole Bible. That's what I do, and I hope and pray that you have or will start a solid, consistent time of reading God's word. I know there are many different read-the-Bible-in-a-year plans, and maybe you are following one, but who cares about how long it takes? Just read it!

I don't listen to audio books, but many of you probably do and find it a convenient way to "read" a book while you're driving, pedaling an exercise bike, or even just spending a quiet evening in your comfy chair. Listening to God's word being read either in an audio book or having someone sitting right with you reading out loud is also a valuable way to get it into your heart, soul, and mind. So if it suits you, do it!

*Studying*

Studying? Not that again! Yeah, studying the Bible, because we need it more than any other thing we have ever studied!

Now, learning to study the Bible can be difficult, but it can be summarized in three basics steps, as described in *Living by the Book*. And by the way, this book is basically "hermeneutics for dummies." —"*hermeneutics*" means the principles and processes of biblical interpretation. Howard Hendricks does a great job in his book of putting this kind of stuff into layman's terms and almost suitable for teenagers as well. But if you want a more collegiate kind of book, Henry A. Virkler wrote a good one called *Hermeneutics: Principles and Processes of Biblical Interpretation*. Either of those books will easily get you on your way to fruitful Bible study. I hope and pray that you will make use of them so that what I'm about to say isn't the only thing you have to go on for Bible study.

So yeah, the three basic steps of studying are (1) observation, (2) interpretation, and (3) application.

Take a pencil, for example. We could probably observe about 100 things about it, but none of those facts by themselves tells us what the pencil *does*—only what it *is*. That is *observation*.

The next step is *interpretation* where we take what we have observed about the pencil and answer these questions: What is the meaning of the pencil? Why was it made? What is its purpose?

After we determine that, step three, *application*, is where we figure out how to use the pencil and how it is meant to work in our life. That is the bare bones of it, and I suppose I could take a whole book to describe it, but since these two guys have already done that, please avail yourself of their books or ones like them.

## *Memorizing*

Quick! Tell me what your best friend's phone number is. Now back in the day, you could have answered that without even thinking, but these days, your phone takes care of knowing that stuff for you. The point is that you *can* memorize things; it's just a matter of whether you need to or really want to.

I love to memorize, partly because I am a very competitive person and I want to "win," and progress, and conquer! Take Psalm 119, for example. That one chapter has 176 verses. Years and years ago, I decided I would memorize the whole thing, and wanted to be able to quote each verse, like, you just say the number and I'll know it. Well, I did that and successfully recited the whole Psalm in order, from beginning to end without looking at it. I won! I conquered! But the most important success was that now I had God's word in my heart, available to the Holy Spirit to bring to mind whenever necessary.

That's the main reason to memorize scripture. As Psalm 119:11 says, "Your word I have treasured in my heart, that I may not sin against You." Yes, I quoted it from memory! But upon checking to be sure I was right, I had to correct *may* from *might*. Anyway, memorizing God's word means we're treasuring it, that we love it, and that we want to keep it within us, and this enables us to more effectively obey it.

So, *how* do we memorize scripture? Well, there are probably books and apps on the subject, so I'll leave that up to you. For me, I just memorize! I don't use any system or strategy. I just do it! One thing is, though, that I memorize whole books of the Bible. I find that memorizing big sections sequentially makes it much easier to remember because the end of one verse leads to the next, and it sort of becomes like one really long verse. And who can't memorize one verse?

One other thing that is important is to get it word perfect according to the Bible version you use. I mean, have you ever been out somewhere talking to someone about the truth of God and tried to quote a verse, only to wind up saying, "Well, it says something like . . ." or "I can't remember where this is but. . . ." Yuck! That's no way to communicate to people how important the word of God is to you! So, memorize word-for-word, which, it just occurs to me, is the way we memorize praise songs. We don't get it "something like" but word-for-word (unless we forget the words all together). The cool thing there is that we don't even *try* to memorize; it just happens by repetition.

And then there is this: I was at a funeral service, and our pastor was speaking and quoting scripture, and as is my habit, like during Sunday sermons, I would kind of quote along with him, whispering the words. So, he quoted a lot during the funeral, and I knew almost all of what he was quoting. But what I didn't know at the time was that one of the people who was there—I think it was one of the funeral home people — was noticing that I was quoting along with the pastor. Someone told me later that this person said to them, totally incredulous, "She knew *every* verse!" To this day, I wonder about what God did with that experience in that person's life.

## *Meditating*

To meditate is to engage in thought or contemplation, to reflect on a certain thing. That requires you to sit still and *think*! I expect that not many in America do that very much. It's all about what's on the screen in front of our faces, whether it's a phone, a TV, or a computer. Everything is coming at us fast, and there is little real thinking or reflecting, but mostly just reacting. It's like a whole necessary process of rationally and objectively assessing that what we are seeing and hearing is replaced with a subconscious, irrational, subjective, and emotion-driven reaction. People who "think" this way can rarely explain their beliefs or even give a good argument for why yours are wrong.

But for me, when the TV is on, I find myself theologically assessing every commercial, like the one that says there is nothing worse than a dead battery. Really? *Nothing* worse? Like maybe losing an arm? Or what really *is* worse than anything is winding up in hell. Or the fast-food chain that says that one of their food items is "value beyond belief." No, what really is value beyond belief is that our Creator sacrificed Himself to give us eternal life. But of course, we're not supposed to be *thinking* anything—just reacting. When my daughter was younger, she'd say, "Mom! Can't you just see a commercial and not say anything? It's just a commercial!" Of course, that statement in itself is theologically incorrect, but I had to pick my battles and eventually kept my comments to myself about commercials (I would still think them, though).

So meditating, at its root, is *thinking*. And as it relates to scripture, it is thinking about what is true about God. And what is true about God is so vast and deep and profound that our puny minds have no end of things to think about Him.

We can meditate or think upon God at anytime and anywhere, not just in a quiet place at the end of the day. Sometimes while I'm driving and seeing the leaves on the trees, and being amazed that Jesus knows how many leaves are on each tree. Then to widen out my perspective and see a forest of them and still He knows the number. And then to think of a world full of trees, and not only that … your mind can travel millions of miles to Mars, and still, He knows every detail, every molecule, and its place. *That's* beyond belief, and yet it's true and certainly worthy of our meditation.

But here, I mean meditation on God's word, and again, there are probably books for how to effectively meditate, but just open God's word and take a verse or short passage. Read it, and then think and think and consider and contemplate and ponder.

I must admit, though, that I am not in the habit of meditating. I don't have a place for it in my intake of God's word. I wish I did so I could expound the awesome benefits of it, but alas … Now I'm just thinking, where could I fit in meditating? Seems good to make it one of the last things I do in the day.

One of my favorite times of the day is at the end of it, after I go to bed. I converse with God and go over the whole day, and then consecrate the next day to Him, seeking His guidance so that I will do what He wants me to. Usually, I just fall asleep still talking to Him or listening to Him. But I'm thinking, how about have a verse or a short section of scripture to meditate on as the last thing I do? I mean, what better way to fall asleep?

Well, you've convinced me! I'll do it! And how about something topical like have verses about peace for the week and about joy for the next week? I think — hey, you know, I'm just remembering that I *did* do meditating years and years ago! I had a small wooden treasure chest. Isn't it right in here? Yes! It's been in this cabinet the whole time. It's about 9 x 7 x 7 inches and is made to look old and worn. And inside—I remember this! I have verses or sections of verses printed on what looks like parchment, about 3 inches wide and of varying lengths and not cut with scissors but torn to make them look old. Man, this is cool! I put a divider in there, and as I go through them, I just pick one out from the left side, meditate on it and then put it in the right side so I don't repeat them until I've gone through all of them.

I guess God just solved my not meditating problem! Anyway, meditate however it suits you. Be still and *know* God.

CHAPTER 4

# We Are Not Our Own

It seems to me that in America we are very entrenched in the mindset of "this is mine and that is yours." Like, I live in *this* house, and you live in *that* one. We put fences around our yards and locks on our doors. Now, this is all well and good because there need to be boundaries, but I think we take this way of thinking too far. At our root, most of us are like children yelling "mine, mine, mine!" about our material possessions, and we likely possess our time just as tightly.

Recently I was waiting at my mom's house for a friend of mine to come and get a couch that was being donated to someone. Knowing I was there just waiting, and being respectful of my time, my buddy texted me and said he would be there in 10 minutes. Without a real thought, I texted back, "No problem. My time is yours." Considering that later, I thought, "Hmm, that's a good attitude to have, I guess."

## God Owns Everything

As soon as you enter the splendorous gates of a king's palace and see the perfectly manicured lawns, the fountains, the exquisite statues, and the groves of fruit trees, you know that it *all* belongs to the king. You approach the palace and see the majestic columns and soldiers stationed at the huge wooden doors that are adorned with painstakingly carved images. You know none of this is yours, and you rightly fear to even touch anything—at least not without permission. So, this world is God's possession. He owns it.

> *For every beast of the forest is Mine, the cattle on a thousand hills. I know every bird of the mountains, and everything that moves in the field is Mine. If I were hungry I would not tell you, for the world is Mine, and all it contains.*
>
> —Psalm 50:10–12

God owns everything because He created it. If we're Bible people, we know this already, but do we really believe it? Do we live like it? Do we *think* like it? For example, being an artist, I was the one who did all the artwork for our Vacation Bible School program. One year, the theme was a jungle setting. So, I used poster board, paint, crayons, markers, hot glue, and cardboard to make cutouts of all kinds of jungle animals, including monkeys, parrots, gorillas, and one majestic jaguar. As opposed to the other animals, this jaguar was photo-realistic, and a little bit bigger than life-size. I intended to keep it after VBS was over. During cleanup, many of the other animals were given to the kids, but when it came to the jaguar, one of the ladies said to the others, "No, that one is Char's. She's keeping it." Now, if we had bought the decorations rather than me making them, anyone could have taken it, but I had the right to it because I made it. And all of the staff honored my right to it. That was about 20 years ago, but I still have that jaguar who I named Gracie. She is sitting right next to my desk here, reminding me of Proverbs 3:21–24 that talks about wisdom and discretion adorning your neck, so I drew some of Gracie's spots to look somewhat like a necklace.

## God Owns Us

A slave is a person who is the property of another and wholly subject to the one who owns them. History shows us and our own consciences tell us that the practice of slavery is wrong. William Wilberforce, a born again Christian and British politician from 1784–1812, led the fight in Parliament for 20 years to abolish slavery. Eventually, on July 26, 1833, three days before his death, Wilberforce heard that the Slavery Abolition Act had passed, effectively ending slavery in the British Empire. Around the world and over the years, many people have fought to abolish slavery, and on the whole were successful with some even giving their lives for it. But why is slavery wrong? The answer can be summed up in the words printed on a medallion created to be used in Wilberforce's campaign. It pictured a black man kneeling, with chains on his wrists and the saying, "Am I not a man and a brother?" Human beings are equal to each other in their nature and therefore have no intrinsic right to rule over one another.

God, however, as our Creator *does* have the right to rule over us, and woe to the one who does not subject himself to that. God rules over the human race, and in a sense, it is His possession, the same as is the rest of creation. Although God owns everything, He doesn't own all people the same way. He only claims personal ownership of the ones He has chosen out of the peoples of the world, having bought and paid for them by His death on the cross. Jesus said this of His disciples:

> *I ask on their behalf; I do not ask on behalf of the world, but of those whom You have given Me; for they are Yours.*
> —John 17:9

Jesus likens those who are His as sheep.

> *I am the good shepherd, and I know My own and My own know Me, even as the Father knows Me and I know the Father; and I lay down My life for the sheep.*
> —John 10:14–15

As "sheep," we are also those who have been adopted by God and are called sons.

*Just as He chose us in Him before the foundation of the world, that we would be holy and blameless before Him. In love He predestined us to adoption as sons through Jesus Christ to Himself.*
—Ephesians 1:4–5

So, God only owns those He has chosen out of the world and given to Christ. Since we are owned, we are also rightly called slaves.

*And having been freed from sin, you became slaves of righteousness.*
—Romans 6:18

Most of the New Testament writers refer to themselves as slaves in the greetings of their letters, although most translations use the word *servant*. As believers in Jesus Christ, we have been chosen by God, bought and paid for by the blood of Jesus, adopted as God's children, and are slaves of righteousness. That should put a healthy perspective on who we really are, but unfortunately—

## We Think We Own Ourselves

Nobody likes a person who acts like they own everything. And worse is when they behave like they own *you*! They have an opinion on everything and are earnest to correct all the "wrong" ways you do things. Unfortunately, some of us are married to people like that, so we know firsthand the effects of someone believing there is no higher authority than themselves. That makes life difficult, not only for the person who gets subjected to them but also for the person themselves. Even though they think they know everything, they apparently don't know enough to be happy because they rarely ever are. It's like children who don't want to subject themselves to the higher authority of their mom or dad, and time-outs or spankings are all too common.

But we must not be too quick to think we don't fit into this category, because we do. Now, there certainly are varying degrees of how much we believe we own ourselves, but it's still there. This belief manifests itself in how we regard ourselves, our money, our time, our abilities, and our material possessions. How do we think about these things? How do we use them? How do we spend them? And not only how, but why? What is our motive? These are necessary questions to ask ourselves, and the answers will tell us where our heart really is and how much we think that what we have is our own.

Years ago, there was a trend to print "Property of" on T-shirts, mostly for schools or colleges. It could say, "Property of Riverdale High Athletic Dept." with an "XXL" thing in the middle. I guess that meant the shirt belonged to the school and must stay in the school or be returned. These days, "Property of" T-shirts say things like "Property of the Jones Family," "Property of My Girlfriend," or "Property of My Hot Boyfriend." These sayings don't imply that the T-shirt itself is the property anymore, but rather the person wearing it. But the statement doesn't match the way the person lives in relation to it. If you called yourself the "property of your girlfriend," then you would necessarily have to live in subservience to her, but nobody does that.

There are also shirts that say, "Property of Jesus," which is literally true of believers. But do we live like it? I saw one shirt that said, "Property of No One," and I think this is probably the most accurate, considering how we really live.

CHAPTER 5

# We Are God's Stewards

Everyone likes a good story, especially in books like this where the author tells some anecdote about themselves to start off the chapter. Well, that's not happening in this chapter. Rather, I'll let scripture tell the tale.

> *For it is just like a man about to go on a journey, who called his own slaves and entrusted his possessions to them. To one he gave five talents, to another, two, and to another, one, each according to his own ability; and he went on his journey. Immediately the one who had received the five talents went and traded with them, and gained five more talents. In the same manner the one who had received the two talents gained two more. But he who received the one talent went away, and dug a hole in the ground and hid his master's money.*
>    *Now after a long time the master of those slaves came and settled accounts with them. The one who had received the five talents came up and brought five more talents, saying, "Master, you entrusted five talents to me. See, I have gained five more talents." His master said to him,*

> *"Well done, good and faithful slave. You were faithful with a few things, I will put you in charge of many things; enter into the joy of your master."*
>
> *Also, the one who* had received *the two talents came up and said, "Master, you entrusted two talents to me. See, I have gained two more talents." His master said to him, "Well done, good and faithful slave. You were faithful with a few things, I will put you in charge of many things; enter into the joy of your master."*
>
> *And the one also who had received the one talent came up and said, "Master, I knew you to be a hard man, reaping where you did not sow and gathering where you scattered no* seed. *And I was afraid, and went away and hid your talent in the ground. See, you have what is yours."*
>
> *But his master answered and said to him, "You wicked, lazy slave, you knew that I reap where I did not sow and gather where I scattered no* seed. *Then you ought to have put my money in the bank, and on my arrival I would have received my* money *back with interest. Therefore take away the talent from him, and give it to the one who has the ten talents."*
>
> *For to everyone who has,* more *shall be given, and he will have an abundance; but from the one who does not have, even what he does have shall be taken away. Throw out the worthless slave into the outer darkness; in that place there will be weeping and gnashing of teeth.*
>
> —Matthew 25:14–30

Let me say first about the third slave who got thrown into the outer darkness: Don't be that guy! This illustrates a person who professes to be a believer in Jesus and likely attends church and does

"Christian" things but is eventually proved to not have true saving faith. This is a serious thing—I mean *really* serious—that a person can believe they are born again and on their way to heaven when they aren't. Jesus said this:

> *Not everyone who says to Me, "Lord, Lord," will enter the kingdom of heaven, but he who does the will of My Father who is in heaven will enter. Many will say to Me on that day, "Lord, Lord, did we not prophesy in Your name, and in Your name cast out demons, and in Your name perform many miracles?" And then I will declare to them, "I never knew you;* depart from Me, you who practice lawlessness."
>
> —Matthew 7:21–23

Jesus teaches that there will be some people who call Him Lord, meaning that they believe they know Him and are submitted to His lordship but will not enter heaven. He foretells that many will say to Him on Judgment Day that they did many things in His name. It might be easy to believe you know Jesus when you have been doing *miracles* in His name, but people who simply congregate with other Christians or do Bible study can also be deceived. The most sobering statement in this passage is Jesus saying, "I never knew you." What we believe pales in comparison to what is *actually true,* so when Jesus says He doesn't know you at the Judgment, that's a terrible spot to be in. That's why scripture pleads with us to:

> *Be all the more diligent to make certain about His calling and choosing you.*
>
> —2 Peter 1:10

> *Be diligent to enter that rest, so that no one will fall, through* following *the same example of disobedience.*
>
> —Hebrews 4:11

> *Show the same diligence so as to realize the full assurance of hope until the end.*
> —Hebrews 6:11

> *Test yourselves to see if you are in the faith; examine yourselves! Or do you not recognize this about yourselves, that Jesus Christ is in you—unless indeed you fail the test?*
> —2 Corinthians 13:5

This last passage states it most plainly, that people can believe that Jesus is in them, that they have Him as their Savior, and yet fail the test. In the end, they are proven to never have known Him at all. Don't let that be you! I'll say with the Apostle Paul, "We beg you on behalf of Christ, be reconciled to God" (2 Cor. 5:20).

So, back to the parable. It describes that the two guys who got the 10 and the 5 talents had a simple job: multiply them! They were required to use what they were given to accomplish their master's purposes, and they did it well. They were faithful and received their reward—entering into the joy of their master.

## That's Mine!

If you have more than one child or know people who do, you've probably heard, "That's mine!" screamed angrily about a toy that both children want at the same time. It may be true that the little blue train was given to Jimmy for his birthday, but really, it isn't anymore his than the floor he's standing on or the roof he lives under. Nor is that house anymore dad's than the earth it sits on. It's easy to say "mine" when we're holding the thing in our hands. And technically, since we went to the store and paid for it, no one else can come up to us and rightly say it is theirs and demand it from us. But neither ought we to withhold it from anyone who asks for it because it is only "ours" through the providence of God that caused it to come to be in our hands.

## The Rich Guy

Imagine if you worked for some rich guy, maintaining his palatial house and grounds. He provides you with a vehicle to go buy mulch and whatever else you need, as well as a credit card to pay for it. Living on the property gives you access to all the rich guy has—a swimming pool, a kitchen filled with all kinds of good stuff, a widescreen TV with stereo speakers, exotic sports cars, and just about anything else you could dream of. And with the rich guy gone most of the time, the temptations to misuse what he has entrusted to you are obvious. I mean, who wants to mow the lawn when it's 95 degrees or skim dead bugs out of the pool when you could recline in the lounge chair next to it and sip iced tea? Or worse, invite your friends over to join you in your depravity for a pool party! The point is that we can't just do whatever we want with the resources God has given us. We must use them to accomplish His purposes.

Hopefully, we all agree that God has given us everything we have and that He has fully supplied us to fulfill His purposes. And further, that we are willing and wanting to follow the example of the two guys in the parable. But it can get really complicated because we have vastly more than a handful of talents at our disposal. Not only do we have to consider how we use our money, but we also have to decide how we will use our time, our abilities, and our material possessions. All these things work in concert with each other, and the complexity and multiple facets of our lives and our inherent belief that all we have is our own will more than likely have us being unfaithful with these resources. The temptation to misuse these things is a great danger, but the greater danger is to misuse them without even knowing it.

## Weird-Sounding Words

Words like *smooth*, *creamy*, *bubbles*, *flowers*, and *kittens* don't sound weird, and maybe that's because they are nice, not weird, things. But there are words that don't sound good at all, even though they are good words. Take *consecration*, for instance, or its root word *consecrate*, which is kind of ugly sounding. It means to declare something sacred or set apart, dedicated to the service of a deity. Then there is the word *sacrosanct*. It doesn't even *look* nice, let alone how it seems like it's two ugly words put into one. I mean, who comes up with this stuff?

Now probably I sound fairly ignorant saying stuff like this, but I am! Although not as much as I was a few minutes ago because I just looked up *sacrosanct*. It does happen to be two (Latin) words put together. *Consecrate* also comes from two words, but I think the *con* part of it is like a positive kind of thing because I'm guessing that the *des* part of *desecrate* is a negative. But what a word—*desecrate*. That's a word that sounds as ugly as its meaning! Anyway, these words are very important when we use them in regard to our possessions. I'm thinking of these words and mainly *consecrate* because it's a word I have begun to use in regard to the plans I make for each day. After I go to bed at night, one of the things I do is go over with God what specific things I want to do the next day. One of those things is writing this book, and I commit it to God, saying, "God, I consecrate this book to You. Lead me and inspire me with what to write, and let it be done according to Your will."

As you can probably tell by now, I am no more qualified than SpongeBob SquarePants to write a book like this, but by God's grace, I am what I am. He moves me to seek Him and has convinced me that I can do nothing apart from Him, so I put everything I want to accomplish into His hands. As much as He enables me to, I trust Him, follow Him, and operate by His power and prompting in me. So, I consecrate everything the night before to God, including the guitar practice I want to do, the pencil drawing I am working on, the novel I am writing, and many other things that I won't say because they may seem too inconsequential to "bother God with," a thing I obviously don't believe *at all*.

The point is that we need to consecrate *everything* to God, even down to the thoughts we think. As it says in Psalm 104:34, "Let my meditation be pleasing to Him." Our thoughts, first and foremost, exist to glorify God, to be pleasing to Him. Think of it. Even our *thoughts* are God's property, given to us to serve His purposes.

> We are *destroying speculations and every lofty thing raised up against the knowledge of God, and* we are *taking every thought captive to the obedience of Christ.*
> —2 Corinthians 10:5

We must really think about what God wants us to do and consecrate everything we have to Him that we would serve His purposes in each of our lives.

## The Other Weird-Sounding Word

When my mother passed away, she left a small inheritance to me. I immediately was prompted as to what I would use most of it for. Believing that it was God's will, I consecrated it, or set it aside, as the funds to publish my novel, if indeed I would self-publish. I considered it *sacrosanct*, that the purpose intended for it was inviolable and beyond criticism, change, or interference. So that money remains set apart for the purpose God intends for it.

Whether we realize it or not, we are constantly consecrating things and considering them sacrosanct. But many times, our motives and focus are wrong. We must be very considerate of what God's purposes are for the time, money, material goods, and abilities He has given us. They are all valuable commodities we have been given to "spend." Now, time and money are things we literally spend, and with time, we can't *stop* spending it. Yikes! Probably we should be more careful with our time than with anything else since we're using it up non-stop!

Thankfully, money isn't tick-tocking its way out of our wallets every second, but we still must be very intentional about how we spend it. It is so with our material possessions, talents, and abilities as well. Obviously, my point is that we need to consecrate everything to God, and when He prompts us to consecrate a certain thing for a certain purpose, we must consider it sacrosanct and not procrastinate, but follow through with doing the thing so as not to desecrate our consecration of it. There! I'm done using all of these weird, ugly words, but I pray that we would do all we can to apply them to everything we have and all we are able to do.

## It All Boils Down to This

The whole point of this book so far can be simply stated: God owns everything, including us, and commands that we be holy, worship Him, and use our time, money, talents, and material possessions to serve His purposes in this world. What His specific purposes are for each one of us is different. But for each one of us as His church in this world, His purpose is the same: to spread the good news of the Gospel. The message we must bring to people is this: God created us to worship Him. But we're born sinners and spiritually dead, so we must be born again through Jesus Christ to receive spiritual life, and thus be reconciled to God, thereby beholding His glory, which brings us great delight. And as this joy satisfies our hearts and souls, we glorify God as we praise Him. Consider these passages:

> *Ascribe to the Lord, O sons of the mighty, ascribe to the Lord glory and strength. Ascribe to the Lord the glory due to His name; worship the Lord in holy array.*
> —Psalms 29:1–2

> *For I proclaim the name of the LORD; ascribe greatness to our God! The Rock! His work is perfect, for all His ways are just; a God of faithfulness and without injustice, righteous and upright is He.*
> —Deuteronomy 32:3–4

> *"Holy, holy, holy is the Lord God, the Almighty, who was and who is and who is to come." And when the living creatures give glory and honor and thanks to Him who sits on the throne, to Him who lives forever and ever, the twenty-four elders will fall down before Him who sits on the throne, and will worship Him who lives forever and ever, and will cast their crowns before the throne, saying, "Worthy are You, our Lord and our God, to receive glory and honor and power; for You created all things, and because of Your will they existed, and were created."*
> 
> —Revelation 4:8–11

We will worship God *forever*. And in the here and now, our whole purpose is also to worship Him, but with the added mission of proclaiming the good news of the gospel to those who do not yet know God, so that through new life in Christ they will become worshipers of God. We must use everything we have and all we do to facilitate worship of God and the proclamation of the gospel. Now, how we each do that is a very individual thing.

> *"For just as we have many members in one body and all the members do not have the same function, so we, who are many, are one body in Christ, and individually members one of another."*
> 
> —Rom. 12:4-6

Some of us will fulfill our roles in a local church as pastors, elders, members of the praise band, or serving in different ministries. From our churches, we send out "missionaries" (I use quotes because technically, we're all missionaries; it's just that some of us all called to different lands and faraway countries). Some support the work of missions by giving monetarily to the church, but no matter what part we play, we are all alive on this planet to spread the good news of the gospel and utilize everything at our disposal to accomplish that.

CHAPTER 6

# Our Bodies and Our Beliefs

When I was 11 and 12 years old, my mom used to say that I was as skinny as a beanpole. Well, she said that about my twin sister, too, and also called us two peas in a pod. I didn't know what beanpoles or pods were, but I liked being "in a pod" with my sister, and I also liked being skinny. And I didn't think much about my appearance back then *until*—until I turned 13 and things started happening to my body. Mainly, it was gaining weight, and it came on suddenly.

At first, it wasn't a big deal to me, but it wasn't long before I started to hear comments about it. After I grew up, I realized that my mom was really fixated on her weight and would always point out other people's body fat levels with contempt (even though she was fairly overweight herself). So, I'm guessing that she was mainly the one who began to tell me I had a "fat stomach." Thankfully, my sister remained a beanpole and didn't have to go through what I did. Anyway, I became really fixated on what my body looked like, and as I gained more weight, I began to feel like some kind of monster was growing on me, coming from the inside out. It was terrible, and I felt helpless to do anything about it. All the ways I had learned to relate to food accelerated this monstrous process.

.

My mom loved to bake, and she was good at it! Her homemade stuff was *so* much better than anything from the store, except for the donuts we got from Buckman's Bakery every Saturday. Looking back, I can see how my mom felt a personal validation of her worth when we ate up the things she baked. I could see this more clearly in later years when she began to overbake things. She couldn't see how they were overbaked, so when I or my sister pointed it out, she got really offended. She probably couldn't allow herself to see or believe that her baked stuff wasn't good anymore because she based her personal value on it being acceptable.

I was clueless about that when I was going into my teenage years. But I had enough perception to see that eating my mom's baked stuff made her happy, and it certainly was easy to swallow. So I ate, and my mom didn't really limit what we could have. It wasn't long before that monster from within emerged and enveloped my whole body and indeed my whole life with a dreadful and unbearable shame about my "fat stomach." I went all the way through middle school and high school feeling terrible about myself and wishing people couldn't even see me. Not unique, I know, as almost all of us have had our hidden shame about one thing or another and our battle with how we regard ourselves.

I was on a bad course of being severely body-conscious, which would plague me for more than half my life. But as I said in the introduction to this book, God transformed my relationship to food by transforming my relationship with Him, which relieved a lot of things. But the "fat stomach" shame was so ingrained in me that it is still "a thing" in my life to this very day. But it is a monster that has been defeated and cut down to size and by God's grace will never rise again.

## These Wretched Bodies!

Almost everybody cares what their bodies look like, but few people *like* what their bodies look like. Some people with lean, beautiful bodies hardly give them a second thought, or else they arrogantly flaunt themselves. Then there are those with fat, ugly bodies or very thin bodies who can hardly stop thinking about them. There are as many opinions and beliefs about the appearance of our bodies as there are people who have them. It seems the majority, though, are those who have more body fat than they like.

Now, I used the term "fat, ugly bodies," and I know that may sound harsh. But having had one, I can say that I was fat, and it was ugly! The worst part of that was that I valued myself based on how I looked, so my estimation of myself was very low. I also assumed that everybody else had the same value system, so I believed everyone had a very low opinion of me as well. Our culture says the same thing, and no doubt that is where my beliefs came from. But really, how twisted and demented is that, to value what a person *looks like* over *who they are*?

Probably I picked up some of this from my mom because she judged people not only on their appearance but also on their mannerisms, even down to the way they chewed gum! It's unfortunate that in this regard my mom was an example of how *not* to be, but I certainly learned that I didn't want to be like that. And I really can't stand it when people make derogatory comments about a person's appearance or mannerisms. It's dishonoring to their personhood, almost as if they aren't even a real person with feelings, hopes, and dreams but only some kind of anonymous cardboard cutout that we sit in judgment over, rendering our score of their acceptability. It's a horrible way to regard people.

## Created, Bought, and Paid For

Are our bodies our own? I think we know the answer to that because we went over it in Chapter 4. God owns everything, and that's because He *made* everything. He created our bodies exactly as He intended each one of us to be.

> *For You formed my inward parts; You wove me in my mother's womb.*
> —Psalms 139:13

Maybe we don't think about this much, but God *created us* and our bodies. He intricately knit us together and chose our hair and eye color, our exact height, our ethnicity, and even our temperament. Billions of people over the centuries, and no two of us alike! Even though my sister and I are twins, we are more different than we are alike. Each of us is a unique, special creation of God, as are our physical bodies that He made for a specific purpose as described here:

> *Or do you not know that your body is a temple of the Holy Spirit who is in you, whom you have from God, and that you are not your own?*
> —1 Corinthians 6:19

Now, the point I was trying to come to with this verse is that we are "not our own." But that really pales in comparison with the statement "your body is a temple of the Holy Spirit." If we really get that, the "not our own" part is almost irrelevant. I mean, imagine if your house was God's temple, all majestic and gold-plated. I don't think we would have to be reminded that it was not our own or that we ought to use it reverently to serve His purposes.

But of course, we're dumb, forgetful sinners, so we need reminding and having things constantly impressed upon us. This passage goes further and says, "For you have been bought with a price." Okay, well, that's even clearer then, that our bodies are not our own. We are *paid for*! But if you're really thinking, you may wonder, *Paid for?* I thought God created us and therefore owns us already?" Well, He did, and He does, but because we were born sinners, we were prisoners, held captive by Satan.

> *If perhaps God may grant them repentance leading to the knowledge of the truth, and they may come to their senses* and escape *from the snare of the devil, having been held captive by him to do his will.*
> —2 Timothy 2:25–26

God had to pay the ransom to redeem us from our sin, and Jesus did that with His own life, shedding His own blood and suffering the punishment we deserved. That is how much He paid to make us His own. So hopefully you have no doubt that you are God's property, and in case we don't understand what we are supposed to do as His possession, the passage in 1 Corinthians that I quoted above finishes with this: "therefore glorify God in your body."

Questions anyone? It's pretty clear, and there ain't no denyin' that we were created by God and then bought and paid for to glorify Him—not just with our hearts and minds, but also with our physical flesh-and-bones bodies.

## Are We Letting Sin Reign in Our Bodies?

So, what does "glorify God in your body" mean? Well, who knows really? But I'll take a stab at it! Probably a good place to start is to look at scripture passages that talks about what we are commanded to do or not do with our bodies. So, I found the following passage to be fairly comprehensive as to how we should regard our bodies. It's kind of lengthy, but I included more verses because of the "therefore" in the middle.

> *Now if we have died with Christ, we believe that we shall also live with Him, knowing that Christ, having been raised from the dead, is never to die again; death no longer is master over Him. For the death that He died, He died to sin once for all; but the life that He lives, He lives to God. Even so consider yourselves to be dead to sin, but alive to God in Christ Jesus. Therefore do not let sin reign in your mortal body so that you obey its lusts, and do not go on presenting the members of your body to sin as instruments of unrighteousness; but present yourselves to God as those*

*alive from the dead, and your members* as *instruments of righteousness to God. For sin shall not be master over you, for you are not under law but under grace.*

—Romans 6:8–14

Because Jesus has conquered sin and death and we have effectively died with Him, we should consider ourselves dead to sin. *Therefore,* we are commanded to not let sin reign in our mortal bodies. Certainly, sexual immorality is a sin we commit with our bodies. Likewise, it is a sin if we punch someone in the face or purposefully break someone's property. But most of us are unlikely to sin in such overt ways.

However, there are things we do with our bodies that we may not have previously classified as sin. Are we letting sin reign in our bodies without knowing it? Before we answer that, it would be good to briefly define what *reign* means in this context. It will be brief because in Chapter 9, we'll get into this much more and consider all the implications and consequences of what it means to let sin reign. Suffice it to say for now that when we let sin reign, it is exerting authority over us the way a king commands his subjects. When we abdicate our authority in this way, we are "presenting the members of your body to sin as instruments of unrighteousness" (Romans 6:13).

But of course, we all do it more often than we like and even more often than we know. So how are we doing it? How are we letting sin reign in our bodies?

I think it's as simple as saying that we "obey its lusts" (Rom. 6:12). An overt example of this would be that if we are working to lose body fat and there is a big, moist, fudgy chocolate cake sitting there, and a voice inside us says, "I want some!" we valiantly resist. But the voice gets louder. "Have some!" If that doesn't work, the voice rationalizes it for us and says, "One little piece won't hurt. Just have a forkful."

If we give in, we have indeed allowed sin to reign, and we have obeyed it. It's really terrible, and I don't like to think of all the years past when I lived like that all the time. But praise be to God for His mercy and patience with us!

So that is an overt and obvious sin, but how do we let sin reign in ways we might not see? I think mainly it's abuse—abuse of our bodies by exercising too much, not getting enough sleep, working too much, eating in an unhealthy way, or any other ways we detrimentally tax our bodies. Now, because of the subject of this book, most of us are probably familiar with unhealthy or gluttonous eating and know well the guilt of that. But less familiar is the guilt we ought to feel when we do too little or too much with our bodies. How much we work, sleep, eat, and exercise can either be abuse of our bodies or not. Whether it is or isn't abuse very much depends on our individuality and our capacities.

I have a list of people I pray for regarding diet and working out. I pray, "May we be faithful to eat and exercise according to Your will for each of us." The "each of us" is key because how I work out and eat is very different from some of the other people on my list. Some think that *walking* is exercise! And for them, according to their beliefs and physical abilities, it *is* exercise. We must really know ourselves because our physical, emotional, and mental capacities are all different.

Now don't get me wrong; I am all for giving it everything I've got and pushing myself to the limit. But the point is that there *is* a limit! For example, I do weight training, and I train really hard. How hard and how often depends on whether I am progressing in size and strength. I know some guys that are at the gym *all the time*. I know that because we used to have to sign in on a card that showed the whole month. One guy's card showed every single day checked! Even Sundays! But guys like this are over-trained and their bodies can't keep up with the amount and intensity of the exercise and so they get nowhere or even regress.

That is abuse of the body and brings me to my next point, that when we detrimentally exceed our capacities, we are abusing our bodies and have crossed the line into sin.

## Why Do We Do It to Ourselves?

So why do some people go the gym every day, get way overtrained and fatigued, and make no progress but *keep doing it*? Or they eat stuff that is bad for them and, worse, consistently eat a lot of it and gain body fat. Or they work too long and hard on a project all day Saturday because they "just had to get it done" (when they really didn't), and then on Sunday they are all worn out and bring much less than their best to teach children's Sunday school. Or someone who overdoes it in the sport of running, and winds up with shin splints or even stress fractures. What goads us to overuse and abuse our bodies like we do? It's simple really, we want what we want and will do whatever we have to do to get it, regardless of the consequences.

Now in one sense, if what we want is good and is God's will, then we dang well better do whatever it takes to get it or accomplish it, regardless of what it costs us. We should give our lives, if necessary. But when we abuse our bodies, we are certainly not acting from such lofty motives. Indeed, we can be sure that our reasons come from a sinful desire to satisfy ourselves apart from God. Let me repeat that. *Our reasons come from a sinful desire to satisfy ourselves apart from God.*

That's why we feel guilt when we eat more than is good for us or when we find ourselves ignoring the voice in our head telling us to put down the hammer and finish the project when we have time. Or turn off the TV, get off the couch, and do the 20 minutes on the exercise bike that we had planned to. But we can be so set on having it our own way that we have successfully deafened our ears to the prompting of God and have disconnected ourselves from our own consciences.

I lived in such a place for years and years, and it was terrible. And I can say without a doubt that I *never* got what I wanted out of *anything* I ever did to satisfy myself. It took decades for God to bring me out of that, and it is only in this last year or so that I have become wholly sold on the truth that my body is not my own but is the temple of the Holy Spirit. I say "wholly sold" because before, I *did* believe that my body was not my own, but I didn't live like it. Now I do. Well, I do *mostly*, but that wretched sin thing.

## Abusing the Temple of the Holy Spirit

I recently got a new-to-me car. It was previously a lease car, and my husband bought it from a dealership that we had bought from for decades. He didn't look it over very carefully when he test-drove it, mainly because he went after work when it was dark, and he also trusted the dealer. It was a super good deal money-wise, so he signed the deal. But when we went back to finish the paperwork and pick it up, I saw it for the first time in the light of day, and all became clear. From a distance, it looked great. But closer up, there were scratches and slight scrapes here and there, and the interior was, well, the person who leased it was a slob. I mean, it was cleaned up, but the evidence was there, especially to me since I am so particular. Thankfully, not long after I had it, a deer ran into the driver's side. The car needed new doors, and the whole side needed to be repainted! So at least that side looked like new! The point is that the person who leased it abused it and didn't care about its condition, knowing that they would be turning it in eventually.

Actually, now that I have written this, it doesn't seem to make the point I wanted to. Well, you know one point that can be made, is that when we consider something isn't really ours, like a lease or rental car, our natural bent is to not take care of it as well. But that is kind of opposite of how we regard our bodies. We possess them fiercely as *ours*! So how come we abuse them like they are rentals?

I mean, on that basis alone, we ought to take good care of our bodies because they are indeed not our own. So how do we dare abuse them as we do? Well, the answer to that we already went over in the previous section, that our physical bodies have powerful appetites, and our sin nature does all it can to goad us to satisfy those desires in unholy ways. We'll get into that whole problem a lot more in Chapter 9.

## Glorify God in Your Body

What does it mean to glorify God in your body? Let's begin by defining what it means to glorify God. I went over that in the middle of Chapter 3, but it's good to reiterate it. To glorify God is to experience Him, to taste and see that He is good (Ps. 34:8), with the outcome that we enjoy Him and are satisfied by Him. Through this experience, we can say that there is nothing and no one better or more desirous than God, nothing more satisfying, nothing that is a greater treasure than He is. This extolling of God for how glorious and all-satisfying He is consummates, or completes, the glorification of Him.

To put it simply, when we love, enjoy, and are satisfied by something, we extol its virtues to all who will listen. It's like being at some event and the sheet pizza gets delivered. People dig in and find it to be the best pizza they've ever had. They enjoy it immensely and are soon very satisfied, but before they are done, they go to those who haven't had any yet and tell them how good it is. More gather around, and the pizza becomes the center of attention and consequently gets all the glory. It gets glorified as the best pizza ever. On an unimaginably larger scale, that is how we glorify God.

So how do we glorify God *with our body*? Let's look again at the Romans 6 passage that we went over in the previous section where we dealt with whether we are letting sin reign in our bodies. We saw that we are not to abdicate our authority over sin and use our bodies to do what is wrong. The passage then says, "but present yourselves to

God as those alive from the dead, and your members as instruments of righteousness to God" (Romans 6:13).

So, that is a good place to start to determine how we glorify God with our bodies. Just do what is right with them! And we must because 1 Corinthians 6:13 says that our bodies are "for the Lord, and the Lord is for the body." It further states in verse 15 that our "bodies are members of Christ." That echoes the truth that we are not our own but that we have been bought with a price. We belong to *God*—heart, soul, *and* body—and consequently we must glorify Him by doing *what is right* with them. Consider the following:

> *Whether, then, you eat or drink or whatever you do, do all to the glory of God.*
> —1 Corinthians 10:31

> *Whatever you do in word or deed, do all in the name of the Lord Jesus, giving thanks through Him to God the Father.*
> —Colossians 3:17

If we combine these commands and apply them to what we do, we must say that we are doing all in the name of the Lord Jesus to the glory of God. Imagine any number of things that you know are wrong to do with your body, but then try preceding those actions with this statement, "In the name of Jesus Christ and for your glory, O God, I do this thing." If we said that every time before we did something, we'd be much more sober and thoughtful about our choices. And yet this is exactly the attitude we are commanded to have.

But let's get back to the important thing—pizza! How do we eat pizza to the glory of God? First off, we're *using our bodies* to eat the pizza, so if we are eating it rightly, we will be glorifying God with our body. When we taste, smell, and chew, we transmit signals to all the gray and white matter, nerve cells, small blood vessels, and fat that are inside our skull, and consequently, we experience mental and emotional enjoyment of the pizza. Now that's using your brain! (and your body). Now, I said we must eat pizza *rightly* to glorify God. As we just saw, we are to do everything in the name of Jesus Christ and for the glory of God. But we can add one more command to that:

> Men *who . . . advocate abstaining from foods which God has created to be gratefully shared in by those who believe and know the truth.*
> —1 Timothy 4:3

We would then have to say, "With a thankful heart, in the name of Jesus Christ and for your glory, O God, I eat this pizza." That's glorifying God when you eat in His presence with thanksgiving to Him for His gift of the pizza and your ability to enjoy it. I spent years and years *not* doing that. I ate under a veil of shame, gripped by the hand of crushing guilt, suffering the absence of God, and helplessly living inside a body I hated. I thought this strategy would actually *work* someday. I mean, how stupid could I have been? But that's what Satan, our sinful flesh, and selfish desires produce.

I think there are many different and much more serious aspects to how we glorify God with our body, such as accepting and suffering illness or injury, keeping ourselves pure from immorality as Paul did with being beaten so many times and Peter did as he was executed. But since this book is about holiness and food, it will suffice to say that we must glorify God in our body by how we eat. We must remember that our body is the temple of the Holy Spirit and that temples are made for worship. So, then, "present your bodies a living and holy sacrifice, acceptable to God, which is your spiritual service of worship" (Romans 12:1).

## Living Sacrifices

What does it mean in Romans 12:1 to "present your bodies a living and holy sacrifice"? What first occurs to me is the story of Abraham going to sacrifice his young son Isaac to God on an altar. If you are not familiar with this, I'll give a short synopsis, but you would do better to read Genesis 22:1–19. The passage says that "God tested Abraham" and asked him to literally sacrifice his young son (about 13 years old) by using a knife to kill him and then burn him on an altar. Abraham proceeded to obey, but at the moment of the knife coming down, God called out and stopped him and said, "Do not stretch out your hand against the lad, and do nothing to him; for now I know that you fear God, since you have not withheld your son, your only son, from Me" (Gen. 22:12).

This happened well before God instituted the Levitical sacrifices of animals. In that system, the animals were killed before putting them on the altar, so they did not need to be bound. But this passage says that Abraham "bound his son Isaac and laid him on the altar" (Gen. 22:9). What must that scene have been like? What was Isaac thinking and feeling? Did he need to be bound because he was fighting and screaming against what he knew was about to happen to him? Mercifully, God instructed Abraham to kill Isaac before lighting the fire. But what if he hadn't? What would the term "living sacrifice" mean then? And in light of this, what does it mean to give our bodies as living sacrifices? First of all, *living* means not dead (obvious, I know), but a sacrifice in the Levitical system was only effective after the animal had been killed and burned on the altar. I think *living* means to *go on* being a sacrifice, to *keep being* one, and to continuously live a life that illustrates God's love and mercy. The following passage illustrates this:

> *Who will separate us from the love of Christ? Will tribulation, or distress, or persecution, or famine, or nakedness, or peril, or sword? Just as it is written, "*For your sake we are being put to death all day long; we were considered as sheep to be slaughtered.*"*
>
> —Romans 8:35–36

Normally, death is instantaneous, but here it is described as taking all day. And it is primarily physical suffering that must be endured "all day." So this sacrificing of our bodies is a lifestyle and must be how we live. Paul says, "I die daily" (1 Cor. 15:31), and in 2 Corinthians 11:23–29, he lists a whole bunch of things that happened to him that included being beaten, shipwrecked, hungry, stoned, cold, sleepless, and in danger from robbers and from the Jews. He ends the section by saying, "Apart from *such* external things, there is the daily pressure on me *of* concern for all the churches" (2 Cor. 11:29).

So, Paul's suffering in this context was primarily external, suffered in his body. He was the prime example of one who gave his body as a living sacrifice, and to such an extent that he could say, "For I bear on my body the brand-marks of Jesus" (Gal. 6:17). To be such a sacrifice, we must relinquish all rights over ourselves, and in this case, it specifies all rights over our bodies. As we have seen, our bodies are not our own. I think these passages teach us to acknowledge that and give our bodies as a sacrifice to God.

We must do what has already been described in this chapter—do not let sin reign in our body but glorify God in our body; use our body as an instrument of righteousness; forego everything that is contrary and obey God by what we do with your body. But submitting our bodies to God is merely a starting point and doesn't really address the aspect of physical suffering or deprivation that we will experience in our day. Paul suffered much in his mission to proclaim the gospel, and while we are on the same mission, it is not likely that we will get stoned or flogged or go hungry. But we all will suffer physically at some point and to some degree, so it is important to know what it looks like to "present your bodies a living and holy sacrifice," at such times.

## The Pain of Being a Living Sacrifice

When we give our bodies as living sacrifices, we are putting ourselves in a position that says we are willing to accept physical suffering.

Many of us know far better than others what physical suffering is, some to the extent of living in a constant state of feeling like we're burning on the altar. This is not a very comfortable thought to offer ourselves to such a condition, but the truth is that when we wholly give our bodies to God, we are in the safest, most soul-satisfying place we can be. That is because when we yield our bodies to God, we are obeying Him, and this obedience is a result of loving Him. And when we love Him, we are filled with joy in Him. But all of this glorious truth can be easily forgotten in the midst of serious pain. Now, I must say that I have never experienced chronic or intense pain—only mild physical suffering. So, it will be difficult for me to write about this knowing that many of you do suffer a lot of physical pain. I pray God's grace to prevail upon you.

## The Value of Pain

We never want pain, but when it comes, it is natural for us to want it to be gone. And we pray, as Paul did, to have it removed. But we must be cautious in this, because there is great value in pain when we receive it as living sacrifices. Though we cannot thwart God's plans, do we short-circuit His benefits to us when we ask for pain to be removed and then He removes it? What may we have missed that we could have benefited from? Think of the number of times you've heard of people going through something very painful and difficult, and when it's over, they say, "I wouldn't have wanted it any different," because of the positive effects it has had. I mean, I pray to be well and healthy and fit, but then I end with "not my will but Yours be done, O God." And you may be thinking that Jesus prayed the same thing when He was faced with the cross, so I guess we are in good company to pray such prayers.

But pain is of great value, and we should wholly embrace what God brings upon us, knowing that He only brings upon us what is the absolute best for us. I'm not saying don't take an aspirin for a headache or don't go to the chiropractor when your back is out of whack, but to have the heart attitude to accept what God brings your way, no matter how difficult it is. Paul illustrates this with his "thorn in the flesh," and though he asked God to heal him from it, he accepted it as being for his good. Consider the following passage:

> *Because of the surpassing greatness of the revelations, for this reason, to keep me from exalting myself, there was given me a thorn in the flesh, a messenger of Satan to torment me—to keep me from exalting myself! Concerning this I implored the Lord three times that it might leave me. And He has said to me, "My grace is sufficient for you, for power is perfected in weakness." Most gladly, therefore, I will rather boast about my weaknesses, so that the power of Christ may dwell in me. Therefore, I am well content with weaknesses, with insults, with distresses, with persecutions, with difficulties, for Christ's sake; for when I am weak, then I am strong.*
> 
> —2 Corinthians. 12:7–10

Now, this response of Paul and how God responds to Paul's request is, I believe, one of the greatest and most important truths in scripture about how we should respond to the pain of physical ailments, injuries, or illnesses. Paul's thorn in the flesh was a physical malady of some ilk, probably a problem with his eyesight, but in the end, Paul boasted or exulted in it. Why? Because it brought about a great spiritual benefit that the power of Christ came to dwell in him more fully than it would have otherwise. Another great thing his pain did for him was to keep him from exalting himself. No matter how great his pain, the spiritual effects of it far outweighed it. This is an awesome thing to comprehend and life-changing when we accept that physical pain is one of the means God uses to bring great spiritual benefit to us.

*And we exult in hope of the glory of God. And not only this, but we also exult in our tribulations, knowing that tribulation brings about perseverance; and perseverance, proven character; and proven character, hope.*
—Romans 5:2–4

The "tribulation" here isn't specifically physical, but it certainly includes it. We see that the suffering results in spiritual growth, and that's the whole point. God's will is that we be made more like Jesus, and He ordains suffering, physical or otherwise, for just this reason.

That is why it is so important to have this matter settled, that our bodies are not our own and that we have yielded them up to God for Him to do as He wills with them. We must never try to override His authority over our bodies by attempting to "heal" them ourselves. I put "heal" in quotes because we are incapable of doing that. We can maybe alleviate some symptoms, but only God can bring about healing and health.

Consider this scenario. A person feels some strange pain they have not felt before and gets worried about it. The symptom just kind of hangs around, and the person, more anxious than before, goes on the Internet and searches for answers. What they find convinces them that there is more wrong with them than they thought, and they make an appointment with their doctor. But the doctor can't find anything of substance to diagnose, and the person goes home thinking that the doctor is wrong because the symptoms are so real. But the symptoms never come to anything and eventually just disappear. I mean, where was God in the consciousness of this person during this whole thing? Again, I'm not saying don't go to the doctor, but don't push God out of the way in an anxiety-ridden effort to get there.

## You Can Quote Me on This

Over the last year or so, and especially in the last three or four months, I have come to regard my body as expendable in my pursuit of spiritual growth and experiencing Jesus more deeply. It's like God has constantly been testing me with this question: Do you trust Me with your body? My answer has increasingly been yes, and to aid me in remaining faithful to this, I have come to have many slogans or mottoes that I tell myself to remind me of the truth of God.

"God, my body is Yours, and the way it is functioning right now is Your will and to my greatest benefit, so I accept it and trust You."

"Jesus, my hope is in You, not in the way my body is functioning right now."

"God, You have me right where You want me."

"God this body is Yours. If I needed it to function differently, You would cause it to."

Following are other pithy statements I don't necessarily quote to myself on a daily basis, but they are nonetheless what I absolutely believe are true.

"We must be willing to expend our bodies, even to death, in the pursuit of spiritual growth and joy in God."

"Our spiritual being is far, far more important than our physical being."

"The spiritual gain far exceeds the physical pain of suffering."

"My body is merely the vessel in and through which God accomplishes His spiritual purposes in my heart and soul."

As such, our bodies are expendable. They may not function as we wish them to, nor look like we want them to, but the thing we can be absolutely sure of is that our *souls* are every moment functioning more as we wish them to and looking more like we want them to. Praise be to God that our progress in becoming more like Jesus is guaranteed.

In the midst of pain, we must *believe* what God says is true and be reminded constantly of it. Many times, I tell myself, "It won't last forever" when I'm suffering with some pain or not feeling well. Even if it goes on to the end of our days, we've got to believe that the span of our life is as short as a vapor breath in the light of eternity. Again, I don't minimize the pain some of you have to endure, but my heart for all of us is that we would trust God with our bodies, that we would believe that everything we experience is meant to increase our humility, our dependence on God, and our joy in Him, with the result that He is ever more exalted in our bodies and glorified by our lives.

One last thing—think of what Jesus had to endure on the cross. It seems that He wished there could be some other way when He prayed to the Father, "Father, if You are willing, remove this cup from Me" (Luke 22:42). But there was no other way to accomplish our salvation, so Jesus said, "yet not My will, but Yours be done."

I have found it very beneficial in the midst of suffering and trial to tell myself, "There is no other way." If there were, God would be doing it that way instead of the way He is. So just remember that the way things are is exactly how God wills them to be because it is for our greatest benefit.

CHAPTER 7

# Our Bodies and Our Effectiveness

My husband and I have some TV programs in common that we like and record them so we can watch them together in the evening. There's something special about watching a program with someone rather than by yourself. There is a certain sharing that goes on, and observations and comments can be made. But when you turn to the other person to say something and their head is back and their eyes are closed, well, that's no fun! Such is the case sometimes, but it happens because my husband has worked all day and is by no means a young guy anymore. Our bodies can only do so much, and when he falls asleep, he has reached a certain limit, and the activity of enjoying a TV program together is over. Thankfully, after a short snooze, he revives, and the program can continue, although at other times, he is just done for the evening.

**The Outer Limits**

Clearly, our bodies have limits. We can only stay awake for so long, lift so much weight, run for a certain distance, concentrate on a computer screen for a certain amount of time, or even eat a certain amount of food, whether too much or too little. When we reach our limit, we are functionally and temporarily disabled from continuing in said activity.

We learn more about our mortality and how helpless we really are, but some of us learn this lesson in a more difficult way than others. You know those sorts of people who just keep going. They don't pace themselves; they can't let go of a thing until they've wrung it out, and then reality brings them to a crashing halt in some form or another. A person like that really doesn't recognize boundaries or time. Seconds, minutes, hours, days, weeks, months, and years are seemingly incoherent to them. What matters is *doing the thing* and getting it done no matter what it takes. It's like a mouse trying to chew a hole to get into a house. It doesn't matter to that wretched little rodent how long it takes, what time of day or night it is, or how much it is annoying the occupant of the house. It just keeps noisily gnawing.

Anyway, seconds and days and weeks and months and years matter because time is the framework in which we operate. These increments are what our internal clocks are set by. The physical benefits of abiding by the constraints of time are numerous, as are the emotional and mental aspects. We say that we *begin* each day, but time didn't stop while we were sleeping. Or we say, "Well, a new month is starting," or we make a big deal about when a new year begins. But nothing is really beginning and ending time-wise. It's all just in our minds.

But it's a good thing that we think in such a manner, that each day is "new," because it gives us the framework to reset and be renewed and refreshed. It also helps us to "start over" when we do something wrong or need to get out of a habitually bad way of living. So, the way we relate to time matters, not only to enable us to start each day refreshed and ready but also to show us when it's time to stop doing something and let up on things that would otherwise become detrimental.

God created time, and He also created its previously described increments. And that is for our good. Time sets boundaries, and the wise person will operate productively within those boundaries when they respect them. Effort is another thing we expend, but it goes hand in hand with how we spend time, so we must be wise and judicious in our use of both.

## The Sky's the Limit!

So why am I talking about limits? Who wants limits? Nobody! But that's how we get into trouble, when we don't limit ourselves or moderate how much effort and time we put into things. We *need* limits—except speed limits. Just take the signs down! People will learn that you can't drive at 100 miles an hour through a small town. I think people would naturally regulate themselves … Oh ho! You disagree? You think we *need* speed limit laws? Well, you're right. We do, but only for those who are foolish, lawless, or have little regard for their fellow man.

> *But we know that the Law is good, if one uses it lawfully, realizing the fact that law is not made for a righteous person, but for those who are lawless and rebellious.*
> —1 Timothy 1:8–9

See? Speed limits are unnecessary for those who are righteous, for those who live according to scripture, who love their fellow man and therefore would never endanger them with fast or reckless driving. That's why I don't usually follow the speed limit because I am not under law but under grace. I follow the *reason* for the law—to keep civil order—but not the letter of the law.

In a similar way, we ought not to live our lives legalistically, setting limits on things just for the sake of it or setting no limits. For example, my brother-in-law proclaimed that since it was June, the furnace shouldn't be on (even though it was only 60 degrees outside and a little chilly in the house). That's kind of denying reality and "keeping the rule," or responding in a manner to how things *should* be rather than how they actually are. So, while we can't run around saying that the sky's the limit all the time, neither should we set artificial, inflexible limits. We must moderate ourselves in a way that is for the good of all and effective to accomplish the goals we have.

## Hangry

No, hangry is not a misspelling, and it's not even a real word. I couldn't dislike it more than I do, but it's a term some people use. It's like when they get really hungry and then get irritable and mad, they call it being—not going to use it again — refer to the heading. Obviously, it is a combination of the words hungry and angry, and those two conditions are so closely related to each other that they can be described as one condition.

But it is a really good example of how our physical condition can affect our emotional and mental state. It can easily compromise how we feel and think and reduce our objectivity. It makes us "see things that are not there" in relationships with other people or in circumstances. We make wrong assumptions about people's motives or actions or read things into a situation that exist only in our imagination.

Then there is the condition of being very tired and how that makes it hard to concentrate on what we're doing. Maybe someone will make two words into one for that too. The point is that our physical condition directly affects our emotional condition and cognitive functions.

### *Carbs and Clear Thinking*

Back before I started keto, when my carbohydrate was relatively high, I experienced how a high-carb intake can negatively affect my memory and clear thinking. I sat down to do my evening scripture review/memorizing time, and I was also (uselessly and hopelessly) dieting, so my calorie intake was low, along with carbs. As I tried to recall a verse, it came easily, much more so than normal, and I thought, "Wow! What goes on?" not having any idea that the low carb situation was the reason. The next night it was the same thing. But I inevitably gave up on the diet, and my carb intake went back up. when I came to memorizing, well, it seemed like someone had stuffed cotton into my brain! No, that would be in my ears ... well, anyway, my brain and ability to recall the verses seemed all muffled. It was then that I thought about the correlation between carb intake and the ability to think clearly. Maybe that's just me, but I couldn't deny the difference.

*Magnesium and Anxiety*

When I started eating ketogenically, I went low on magnesium fairly quickly, but without knowing that that was the problem. I soon figured out by searching online that the muscle twitches I was having were from salt, potassium, and magnesium being out of balance.

I had been very anxious and on edge during that time as well, and once I started supplementing with magnesium, the muscle twitches cleared up as did the anxiety. But what I found out later was that the anxiety, restlessness, and crazy swings of emotion had almost everything to do with low magnesium.

Since I prefer to get all my nutrients from whole food, I cut back on magnesium supplements, emphasizing foods richer in magnesium, but I soon started with anxiety again. Resuming my regular amount of magnesium supplements cleared it up, but was it a placebo effect or not? You be the judge, but I believe there was a clear correlation.

Another thing I learned was that feeling anxious based on purely the physical factors of my body being out of balance predisposed me to worrying about things. It's like, my *body* was anxious, so my *mind* naturally went along with that and decided there were things I should worry about. For those of us who deal with anxiety, we don't have any problem turning things into problems that we can worry about that aren't really problems at all. When our body is helping us do that, it can be overwhelming.

The worst part of a situation like this is that anxiety is a real indictment against the sufficiency of God. To put it plainly, anxiety is sin, not only because it violates the biblical mandate to not be anxious but also because anxiety says, "God, I don't trust You with this situation. I don't believe that it is for my good." Nobody wants to be saying that to God, so at the least we should manage our bodies and be as healthy as we can be to minimize how our physical condition negatively affects our emotional and spiritual condition. I'd like to go into this more, but John MacArthur wrote a good book called *Anxiety Attacked* that will tell you all I would like to and more.

## Barometers

Last night, right before I went to sleep, this phrase popped into my head: "Are our bodies our barometer for happiness and peace?"

I woke up this morning (earlier than usual — it's only 5:30!) and am sitting here trying to explain what the point is. I don't really know what a barometer is, so let me go look it up. Okay, so, barometers measure air pressure, and people use them to forecast the weather. When it is a sunny day and the air pressure falls, rain is on the way. I was just watching a video to learn this and noted that the guy said, "When the air pressure falls, bad weather is on the way." By saying "bad" weather, I assumed he meant rain, so high pressure means "good" weather like sun and blue skies. The lower the barometric pressure, the "worse" the weather is, like severe thunderstorms.

So, our bodies don't have a barometer, but I think our minds do in relation to our bodies. When our bodies are not functioning correctly, it is natural to be concerned, and most of us will start to worry when we don't know what is going on. Our emotional pressure changes, and the clouds of anxiety descend. We look for answers, but during this time of not knowing, our anxiety can run high, especially for those of us who are overly concerned with the condition and health of our bodies. Now, I mean this in a hypochondriac kind of way where we are preoccupied with a certain physical symptom that feels like something is "wrong." And when it is something unknown or previously unexperienced, we can begin to give it an inordinate amount of our attention. This obviously disrupts our peace, and as long as we are experiencing the unknown symptom, our barometer will be telling us that we should be experiencing a downpour of anxiety and worry. But is this how we should respond?

Since I am apparently a hypochondriac, God has been giving me much fodder in this last year to overcome that malady by giving me minor intermittent physical symptoms that get my attention and set the stage for me to worry. Like my right pinky finger will sometimes feel numb on the end, or my left ear sounds funny when I'm chewing something, or around my right eye there is a funny feeling like a tiny little muscle twitching, or I'll just all of a sudden feel really sleepy and can hardly keep my eyes open (like right now actually). All these things are random and just come and go. In addition, my transition into eating ketogenically had my health seriously compromised because I lost too much weight too fast, which almost put me in the hospital.

So, I've had a lot of room for anxiety, but is it justified? To put it simply, no. But I think we live like it is. I believe that in part we have made our happiness and peace depend upon how our bodies feel. But we can't really control our bodies, so do we want to make our emotional stability depend on their condition?

## Recalibrating the Barometer

Another thing I learned about barometers is that they have to be calibrated to the geographical area they will be used in. The readings will be off if the barometer is not calibrated to the local and current barometric baseline. I am sure that the weather guys on TV are very careful with that since they have a hard enough time getting accurate weather forecasts.

So, we too must be careful to calibrate our happiness barometer to the right thing. As we have just seen, calibrating it to our ever-changing physical condition is foolish. Scripture is clear that the anxiety this will produce is a sin and an indictment against God's love for us. Consider the facts that God owns our bodies, dwells within our bodies, sustains our bodies, and uses our bodies to accomplish His will. The importance of our bodies to God cannot be overstated because He uses them to achieve His perfect plan for each of our lives.

I believe He will never allow or cause our bodies to be in any condition other than what is most effective for accomplishing His goal and what is to our greatest benefit, even when it is illness, injury, or something we think is wrong with our body. So let us pray, "God, You have me right where You want me. My body is Yours and is exactly as it needs to be for You to accomplish Your purpose. I wholly accept how I feel and trust that this is for my good and Your glory." And let the barometer for our happiness and peace be on the rock-solid foundation of the One who always does everything for our good and who never changes.

## Our Bodies and Our Productivity

I have some strange malady that renders me physically inoperative for two or three days at a time. The doctor doesn't have an answer, but I'm not much interested in one because the only thing they could possibly do is suggest some kind of medication where the side effects are likely worse than the supposed "cure." And I already eat as well as I can, am diligent with physical exercise, and am wholly committed to spiritual health and growth. Anyway, I just suffer through these spells of not feeling well. I have to lie down and be still. My appetite disappears, my energy goes to zero, and I am sleeping or snoozing for at least a day and a half. Once it's over, I go back to normal. The point is that *I accomplished nothing for two days because my body was not functioning correctly.*

Similarly, when we get the flu, suffer a migraine, break a leg, strain our back, or slice our hand open, we become limited in what we can accomplish. Now, getting sick or being injured can't really be helped, but there are other ways we become limited that we inflict on ourselves. The two main things being not getting enough sleep and not eating in a way that promotes good health.

I am not going to say that we need a healthy body to be effective in accomplishing God's will for our lives. Certainly, many of us labor successfully while being in poor health, some for years and years. But as far as it depends on us, we should seek to be as healthy physically as we can be. I believe that the healthier our bodies are, the clearer our thinking is, the more stable our emotions are, and the more productive we are overall.

## Love Your Body

If we're convinced that we ought to be as healthy as we can be to optimize our spiritual and emotional functionality, what must our motivation be? Well, we can start with love because if you don't love something, you don't take care of it. Okay, so an example, I watch a reality show called *American Pickers*, and there are these two guys who travel the country looking for antiques and what they call "rusty gold." They buy this stuff to sell in their stores. I can't tell you the number of times I have seen these guys look at rusty cars just sinking into the earth as they sit there and rot and rust, dying a death that takes years, and yet the owner of the car doesn't want to sell it because he "loves" it. What?! Really? That's how you treat something you *love*? One of those cars sat there so long that it had a good-sized tree growing up through where the back window used to be. On the other hand, I have a Harley Davidson Sportster motorcycle that was 11 years old back in 2020. A couple weeks ago, I was hanging out at the local H-D dealer, and a guy who was there said, "Wow, that looks great. What year is it, a 2017?" I said, "No, it's a 2009 with 35,000 miles on it." He was dumbfounded, and I replied, "You know why it looks that good? Because I *love* it, verb form of love." In other words, I take really good care of it.

Some may object to the matter of loving our bodies, like it's vain or narcissistic. But when I say *love* our bodies, I mean to treat them well, to provide for their needs, and to not abuse them. It's like how we love people. When they are hungry, we feed them; when they are cold, we invite them into a warm house.

But of course, as we know, love is doing more than your duty to love. It is delighting in doing it and also delighting in the object of love. Usually, it's another person, but when we try to apply this to ourselves, we get a little squirmy (another weird-sounding word, but I won't go into it). Scripture is clear that we naturally love ourselves, and indeed *commands us* to love ourselves. Squirmy again? Consider this:

> YOU SHALL LOVE YOUR NEIGHBOR AS YOURSELF.
> —Matthew 19:19

Don't gloss over the "love yourself" part of it. Just like we love (verb form) our neighbor by how we relate to them and what we do for them, so we should love ourselves the same way. I say we "should" because we usually don't, not consciously anyway. But scripture clearly assumes that we *do* love ourselves. If we didn't, Jesus would not have commanded us to love our neighbor *in just the same way* that we love ourselves. Now, this is a whole other thing, our relationship with ourselves, and it could be a whole other book, but thankfully, it's part of this one in an upcoming chapter, so stay tuned!

> *So husbands ought also to love their own wives as their own bodies. He who loves his own wife loves himself; for no one ever hated his own flesh, but nourishes and cherishes it.*
> —Ephesians 5:28–29

Whoa! How do you get around all that, if you think it is narcissistic or arrogant to love yourself? This says that a husband is to love his wife *as* he loves his own body. Clearly, it is assumed that he loves his body. The passage emphasizes that by stating that no one hates their body but on the contrary loves and nourishes it. A further point is that the one who loves his body, loves himself. We see this in the statement that "he who loves his own wife [as he loves his body] loves himself." There is so much in this passage, but suffice it to say, we must love our bodies because no one truly hates their body. We actually nourish it and care tenderly for it. So, you love yourself; get used to it and start acting like it!

## When Love Looks Like Hate

The idea that we love our bodies and tenderly care for them hardly seems true when we see people abusing their bodies with alcohol, drugs, food, and a host of other ways. When we see a heroin addict, their body emaciated, eyes sunken and vacant; an alcoholic with liver and cardiovascular disease; or someone who is suffering the effects of obesity with diabetes, joint pain, heart disease, and many other complications, we don't see someone who is *loving* their body. It's more like they are hating their body by abusing it, and in some respects, that is true. But how this fits into the truth that we actually love our bodies is explained by our inherent sin nature. Ever since the fall of Adam and Eve, mankind has been seeking to satisfy themselves by whatever means they desire. And apart from faith in Christ, it will always be the wrong way, with negative consequences. This is because our sin nature corrupts *how* we try to be happy.

As we saw in the early chapters of this book, true happiness is only found in worshiping God, which produces joy in Him and Him being glorified as all sufficient. Any other way fails because all other attempts at happiness have the wrong object. That explains the one thing the previous examples of the addict, the alcoholic, and the obese person have in common—excess. They all, along with any other overindulgent use of the body, do not find true satisfaction in what they do and unfortunately believe that more of the same will eventually work. It is a tragic thing, but we see the veracity of it in people who are slowly killing themselves with their corrupted attempts at happiness. I certainly was on that path until God saved me from it. He is indeed the only means by which we can be saved from our lives of excess.

Imagine if you were two people trying to lose body fat, so you committed to no chocolate cake for a month. But one of yourselves puts a piece of cake in front of you and says, "Don't you want it? I know you do." But your other self resists. "No!" So, then an argument starts, and it goes back and forth, getting heated. Now, right off, it is plain that your two selves are not acting in a loving way, especially the bad tempter self. The fight goes on, but eventually, the bad self forces the good self to eat the cake. That's not loving.

We've all been there in one way or another, doing what we don't want to do. It's the *opposite* of love. Imagine if a real person forced you to eat cake and even showed up every day to make you do it until you were actually gaining weight. That's not love, man!

So, when I say that we must *love* ourselves, I mean we must do what is the best for us because that's what love does. That's what God did when He sent Jesus to save us—because He *loved* us. He did what was best for us and gave us spiritual life so we could know Him and worship Him. That's love.

## Honoring the Temple

How do we set limits, break out of excessive behaviors, and truly love our bodies? You probably have a clue from the heading for this section. As we have seen, our bodies are the temple of the Holy Spirit, owned by God but managed by us. That is a huge responsibility, but thankfully, we are not left on our own to manage ourselves and take care of our bodies. God works in us, accomplishing His will (Phil. 2:13), so we can depend on Him to enable us. Yet we are not left with nothing to do. Paul says of himself, "But I labored even more than all of them, yet not I, but the grace of God with me" (1 Corinthians 15:10).

We've got to get to work and fight hard, but all the while depending on God and being carried along by His power. But this is not an easy place to get to. You have to experience it to believe it. And it is not something you just start doing, like flipping a switch. It is *God* who is at work in you, and it is *His* grace that enables you. So, it is up to Him as to how and when He brings that to bear in your life, but with all your heart, pray for that enabling. Being empowered by God like this is really the heart of the matter and our success in winning the fight to truly love our bodies and honor them as God's holy temple. That's what Chapter 9 is all about. So for now, I hope to convince you that honoring your body as God's temple is the place to start and the way to go.

## Holy in Body and Spirit

Scripture talks much about being holy in our spirit and our hearts and minds, but it also mentions being holy in and with our bodies.

> *The woman who is unmarried, and the virgin, is concerned about the things of the Lord, that she may be holy both in body and spirit.*
>
> —1 Corinthians 7:34

## OUR BODIES AND OUR EFFECTIVENESS

To be holy in body is really no different than to glorify God with your body, which we just went through in Chapter 6. But another aspect this passage teaches us is that being holy in body takes concerted effort. We must *focus* and be diligent!

Certainly, we don't have to be unmarried to do this, to be concerned about the things of the Lord. But being unencumbered by a spouse and children makes it much easier to focus. Though I am married, my husband is super low maintenance—and I mean *super low*. It's like living with a very nice roommate who never leaves a mess or asks for anything. So, I have my time to myself, and since I don't work, I am free to do what I want when I want! But of course, writing this blasted book is taking a lot of time, so you'd better make it worth my while and get with the program!

Seriously, though, we all have the time and focus we need to be "concerned about the things of the Lord" because I can't imagine that God wouldn't provide that. If we feel like we just don't have the time, it's more likely that we have taken on more than is God's will for us to do—but that's a different book.

Anyway, the intended result of being concerned about the things of the Lord is that we would be holy, not only in spirit but in body. The word *body* here literally means a physical body, and as we have seen, there are many things we can do with our bodies that are unholy. We must do what is holy and right with our bodies, and we will do well to follow Paul's example.

> *But I discipline my body and make it my slave, so that, after I have preached to others, I myself will not be disqualified.*
> —1 Corinthians 9:27

Paul related to his body as a master to a slave and made it his servant. His body served his purposes, not the other way around. He did that so he would not prove himself to be a hypocrite after he had preached the word of God. He was saying that the way he lived and the way he treated his body were congruent with his message. So we must do likewise, but it can prove to be very difficult. Many times, we let our bodies be our masters, obeying their commands for more and more. I mean, the facts of the Christian message, when lived out, ought to have us living disciplined, peaceful, joy-filled lives where we do what we know is right. But even Paul did what he hated, so surely there is hope for us!

Chapter 9 awaits to help us understand how to effectively fight this battle to do the good and right thing. But for now, the next chapter will graphically illustrate the bad and wrong things we do in our relationship with food.

# CHAPTER 8

# Our Food and Our Fidelity

Now we really come to it. After all that has been said about how holiness equals happiness, that we are not our own but belong to God, that we are His stewards of our bodies, that we must love our bodies and glorify God with them, we now come face to face with what is for most of us our biggest problem with living according to these truths—our relationship with food. As I have been writing this book and have talked about it with others, I have often referred to it as "the book on food and holiness." And that is exactly what it is. Of course, you know that because I have referred to our relationship with food throughout it so far, but this is where the going is getting tough for some of us. Grab onto those bootstraps and—well, actually, that's useless because we can't pull ourselves up, so grab onto God and get ready for—

## A Pie in the Face!

If you're like me, you're wondering what flavor the pie is. Banana cream? Lemon meringue? Key lime? Now, I wouldn't mind a pie in the face if it was a really good pie because then I could eat what was stuck on me. But most often, it's just a pan of whipped cream, so that's no fun. Anyway, let's get serious about this food thing and be willing to really see what is going on inside ourselves.

I hope you're going to feel a pie in the face about your relationship with food. You'll be surprised, appalled, and annoyed, and then have to clean a mess off of yourself. But you will suddenly see things about yourself that you never have before and be appalled at the sinfulness of it and annoyed at the mess you now have to clean up.

Well, *you* won't clean it up, *God* will, but you'll have your end of the bargain to hold up as well (by God's power and grace, of course). So, I pray that you will truly see and accept the reality of how you relate to food and that you will wholly yield yourself up to God. I pray He will empower you and set you free from a sinful relationship with food and bring you into a holy relationship with it where pure enjoyment and genuine satisfaction can take place.

## "Just the Facts, Ma'am"

I'm not old enough to remember seeing that old detective show on TV where the detective said, "Just the facts, ma'am, just the facts" when he was trying to solve a case. But I sure understand why he said it. He wanted just the pure facts of what happened, not how a person felt as a witness to crime or what the whole thing meant to them or whatever. All that emotion and editorializing can really muddy the waters of the facts, so to tell just the plain facts first gives a much clearer picture of reality.

We must have as accurate an understanding of reality as possible to most effectively overcome sin in our lives. We need to see and know the truth and comprehend the bare facts of our situation. We need an objective, unemotional description of our actions. I hope I have emphasized this enough because we can so quickly rationalize the facts of our wrong behavior to the point that we actually change the facts into "facts" that exist only in our imagination. It's like a saying from this guy on a TV program where they were trying to disprove scientific myths about things. He would say, "I reject your reality and substitute my own." Kind of humorous, but when we do it for real, we get into all kinds of trouble. And we've all done it, rationalizing doing something that we know we really ought not to do.

We actually have to *talk ourselves into* eating that chocolate chip muffin instead of just a banana. I mean, we argue with ourselves to do the *wrong thing*! Really? Like a court case, the defense presents all the reasons why it's okay to eat the muffin while the prosecution gives all the facts about how it is wrong. As we have experienced, the defense often wins, even though everyone knows the argument was flawed.

Our sin nature runs so deep that its sick desire to satisfy itself in unholy ways can overwhelm our emotions and completely derail our rational and logical grasp of what is truly right. Truth matters. Facts matter. Have I made the point?

Maybe you can see that I'm building up to something, setting the stage to get you in the right place and trying to soften the edges a bit. Well, you're right. I am. This is because I want you to be as objective and unemotional as possible, to receive the truth I am about to share, for fear that you will not receive it at all.

## The Sanctity of Marriage

What? Marriage? Are we still in the right book? What does that have to do with food and holiness? Everything, really — not marriage per se but the fundamental basis of marriage—the commitment two people have made to each other and the resulting covenant that exists between them. Now, stick with me, I'll keep this brief, but the point I want to make is critical and necessary to everything else I will say in this book.

Aside from our relationship with Jesus, there is no relationship in the world more sacred, more intimate, more meaningful, or more satisfying than a godly marriage. Consequently, there is no relationship that has more capacity for desecration, betrayal, and pain than such a marriage that has been violated by unfaithfulness. Unfortunately, most of us have had experience with this, whether we were the victim, the perpetrator, or the family member or friend who helped somebody through it. I think the emotional trauma that happens to the betrayed spouse is so severe because the reality of marriage is so profound. Consider this:

*So they are no longer two, but one flesh. What therefore God has joined together, let no man separate.*
—Matthew 19:6

The two not only become one, but they become one *flesh*. God declares that the two are *one body*. How can this be? After marriage, there are still *two* people. It's miraculous really, but maybe not so much when we understand that it is God Himself who has joined them together.

Now, maybe we think that this only means that God providentially brought a man and a woman together through certain circumstances, that they stood before God, pledged their commitment to each other, and then the minister pronounces them husband and wife. While all of that is true, God's "joining" them goes much deeper and more seriously than that. Surely there is a relational and emotional joining, and in some sense, the physical joining consummates the marriage. But I think the most important aspect is the spiritual joining that God Himself does. It is *His* decision and an act of *His* will that brings a marriage into existence.

When a man and woman say, "I do," they're not only agreeing with each other but with God as well. They may not consciously do it or even have a relationship with God, but He observes their promises made to each other and holds them accountable to that. It's kind of like this: imagine a fenced-in field with a herd of oxen in it. Two of the oxen really like each other, and they come before Farmer Brown. One ox, Big John, says, "We want to work together."

And Daisy agrees, saying, "Yes, we want to be the pair you use." So, Farmer Brown agrees, puts a yoke on them, and hooks them up to his wagon. The farmer joined them together with the yoke so that they are effectively one ox. There was an agreement between Big John and Daisy, but when the farmer joined them together, there came to exist an agreement between the three of them. The oxen have made a lifelong commitment to walk with each other under the yoke of Farmer Brown and to not only be faithful to the covenant they have with each other but also to the covenant between them and the farmer.

## Keeping the Covenant

Marriage is an illustration of Christ and us, His church. We are called the bride of Christ, and when we were born again, we received the Holy Spirit as a pledge guaranteeing our inheritance in Christ and our being part of the marriage supper of the Lamb (Rev. 19:7–10). Because Jesus is our husband, we must be faithful to Him above all else.

Because Jesus is also our God, everything we say, do, and think must be oriented around Him. One of the Christian musicians I like has a song that says, "I don't want to make a move without You." I couldn't agree more. Every move, every decision we make must have at its heart the desire to do God's will. We must consecrate ourselves to this and not make a move without God.

This means that if we are seeking to do God's will, we are seeking *Him* and asking Him to show us what He wants us to do. That is good and right because as His servants and stewards of all we are and all we have; it is only natural for us to look to Him to tell us what He wants us to do. Agreed? I hope so! Really, this puts us in the best possible position for making decisions about what we should do.

If we are getting our instructions from the God who knows the end from the beginning and only does what is absolutely best for us, we ought to listen and follow wholeheartedly! Considering this, when we decide on a course of action, we must be as sure as we can be that it is God's will and that we are depending on God to empower us to see it through to the end.

I shared in the introduction of this book how, in a desperate attempt to get free of my addiction to sugary foods, I made a commitment to God to never eat refined white sugar again. It was a test right from the beginning. Did I love God more than food? I can't tell you how many times I said, "God, I love You more than these Oreos or more than this chocolate mocha ice cream." And there were not only those tests just between me and God, but so many times I'd be at a ladies' social at church or at someone's birthday party and have to say no to the cake or cookies. It was not comfortable, especially at church where I felt the sting of disapproval from some who thought I was being "too extreme" or inflexible, and legalistic.

The most difficult test was my wedding cake. I had my mom make it using no sugar (don't remember what she used as a sweetener), but that got a lot of flak from most everyone. I took it, though, and maintained my "God, I love You more than food." In this case, it was "God, I love You more than what people think about me." I mean, that's really what it comes down to. Do we love God more than what we want to eat, and do we love Him more than what other people think about our commitment to how we eat? Our covenant is with our *God*, not food or other people, and we must be faithful to that covenant, no matter what.

## Breaking the Covenant

Remember the oxen, Big John, and Daisy? Imagine that a few years after being yoked together Daisy becomes disgruntled with Big John. She complains to Petunia, one of her pasture buddies, "He's just not pulling his weight anymore, and he's gotten kind of fat and soft, probably because I'm doing almost all the work!" "I can see what you mean. Glad I never got married," replies Petunia. Daisy labors on, feeling she should keep her commitment. But one day Petunia says, "How long are you going to keep doing all the work with that big fat cow?" Something snaps in Daisy, and she finally leaves Big John for a new, young ox named Apollo that she has had her eye on.

We do the same thing with Jesus when we abandon the commitment we have made for how we will eat. Like, if we decided not to eat any dessert for a week but then halfway through the week, we start to not like it very much and say to ourselves, "Well, I made the no-dessert rule, so I can break the rule." This is true in a sense, but we have also made this commitment with our God. If He led us to commit to "no desserts this week," then we cannot "unyoke" ourselves from it just because a salted caramel cheesecake is calling to us.

Our relationship with Jesus requires us to keep our word, even when we have lost enthusiasm for it. We are yoked with Him, and consequently we walk the same path, and if it is the path He wants us on, we can't just arbitrarily turn aside from it. To leave it is nothing short of committing adultery against Jesus with our food god.

Think that's too extreme to see it that way? If you do, I don't know what else you would call it. I mean, it's plainly being unfaithful, which is what adultery is. I believe it's that serious. And what's even more serious is how easily we gloss over what we are actually doing and, worse, how often we engage in it. This is a stark reality, and we will try to rationalize somehow that it isn't. But it's no different than what God condemned the nation of Israel for in many, many places in the Old Testament.

> *Yet they did not listen to their judges, for they played the harlot after other gods and bowed themselves down to them. They turned aside quickly from the way in which their fathers had walked in obeying the commandments of the Lord.*
>
> —Judges 2:17

This clearly teaches that God considered Israel a harlot when they turned from Him and valued other gods as more important. Does the salted caramel cheesecake mean that much to us that we would turn aside from the way in which we had committed to walk and forsake our God?

## Weak as Water

It's a sad thing that we can so easily devalue and dishonor God and exalt food, and it should grieve us to the depths of our soul. But it's a reality that we struggle with, and we are indeed "weak as water" to fight temptation. Water is weak in the sense that it is helpless to do anything other than conform to the shape of the place it occupies. Apart from God, we are just as weak to do anything other than conform to the desires of our sin nature. Thanks be to God that He knows our frame, that we are but dust, and that His sufficiency is enough for us to overcome any temptation!

This is easy to say, but we all know the grisly reality of failing again and again. But take heart. In Chapter 10 we'll get into how to live in the power of God and experience success more and more often. For now, though, I want to look at food—what it is *for* and whether there is such a thing as "holy" and "unholy" food.

CHAPTER 9

# Food and Our Definition of It

You know me by now, that I like to start at the root of things and come up through a strong foundation to build my case and make the point. So, let's start in the root cellar. "What is food for?"

That might seem like a dumb question, but how would you answer it? Some might be dopey and say, "It's for eating." Others will say, "It's for enjoying," or "It's to comfort us." All of that is true. Food *is* for enjoyment, but first and foremost we know that food is for fueling our bodies. The same as gasoline fuels a car, our bodies need calories to operate. We need the macronutrients of carbohydrates, fat, and protein that contain enough micronutrients of vitamins and minerals to optimally fuel, feed, and maintain our bodies. It's simple, but it would be even simpler if we were like lions.

The female lions go out on a hunt, manage to take down a big water buffalo, and then the rest of the pride comes and digs in, eating until their little tummies are full and round. Then they head for their favorite napping area and lie around for a couple of days before they get hungry again. No fuss, no muss. No overeating, no arguing with themselves about eating fewer fatty eyeballs and trying to eat the leaner meat on the legs or chastising themselves for not eating more salad. Lions have it easy, because they don't have a sin nature that goads them to excess. Wolves don't either. They hunt down a moose, eat only what they need, and leave the rest for later. You never see a fat lion or a wolf with heart disease or diabetes that was brought on by poor eating.

If we could just primarily approach food with the fundamental and core belief that it is for fuel, we would be a lot better off. But that would be too easy, and for many of us, we have spent all our lives in a spiritual and emotional battle with food. Many times, we see it as an enemy that we are almost inextricably entangled with, and we need to see a way out. Thanks be to God, there is a way out, and He will bring us through by showing us how to be more like lions and wolves!

## What Is Food?

Think this is a dumber question than "What is food for?" Consider a fresh, ripe strawberry or a strawberry-flavored gummy bear. Or take corn on the cob with a side of cheddar cheese compared to a bag of cheesy corn puffs. They have similar ingredients, but which is really food?

It's amazing what America has created and put in front of our noses and proclaimed to be food. As a country, we've bought into all of it and are suffering the consequences of it. It's no wonder that one in two people in this country is pre-diabetic and that so many people suffer with physical ailments that are the direct result of not fueling their bodies with enough nutrients. As a society, we also overfeed ourselves with garbage "food," which causes us to carry excess body fat while at the same time actually being malnourished. And we not only do this to ourselves, but our kids learn our bad habits as well. Even many of our pets suffer the same fate of being overweight and unhealthy.

So, what is food? I think there are as many definitions of that as there are people who would define it, but we can probably all agree on a couple of categories—whole food and junk food.

Let's take junk food for instance. It hardly needs defining because we know what junk is and what it means. It's anything that is worthless, meaningless, or has been discarded as trash. Things that no longer function correctly can also be termed as junk.

Imagine that you run out of gas in your car and walk to a farm, find the farmer, and ask if he has any gas. He says no, but you see a big gas can sitting there and ask about it. He says, "Well, there *is* gas in there, but it's been sitting there for years, so it's junk." At your insistence, he gives it to you because you figure gas is gas. You take it and put it in your car, but it won't start. That's because gasoline chemically breaks down and will no longer function if it sits too long. So, your car won't start, the gas tank is contaminated with the bad gas, and you wish you had taken the farmer's word for it that the gas truly was junk.

But we gladly put junk *food* into our bodies! Why? Well, we all know why. It's because it tastes good, and we greatly enjoy eating it! I think the Apostle John had an idea of what this was like. "I took the little book out of the angel's hand and ate it, and in my mouth, it was sweet as honey; and when I had eaten it, my stomach was made bitter" (Rev. 10:10). Seriously though, it tastes good going down, but then our poor bodies have to try to process it and deal with the consequences. Our blood glucose levels rise as the junk food gets metabolized. Much of it immediately gets stored as body fat because it contains almost nothing that meets our nutritional needs. On the other hand, whole foods go into our system and get efficiently processed with all the nutrients being shuttled to various locations to meet our body's needs. No fuss, no muss!

## The Good, the Bad, and the . . .

If you're old enough or a fan of Clint Eastwood's cowboy movies, you know the next word in the heading of this section because it's the title of a spaghetti Western made in 1966. It starred Eastwood as the good guy, Lee Van Cleef as the bad guy, and Eli Wallach as the ugly guy. Now, this doesn't have much to do with food except that it makes for descriptive categories.

In the previous section, I described food as "whole" and "junk," but those are at opposite ends of the spectrum. There is a space in the middle for merely "bad" food. For example, an orange is a whole food, which is good. Orange juice, which is more in the middle, is bad. Orange popsicles are, well, just ugly—at least from your body's point of view. You may love orange popsicles or, better, those amazingly delicious orange creamsicles, but your body doesn't like them at all. The problem is with our taste buds and emotions. Some of us are absolutely ruled by these two things, driven on by our sin nature's unquenchable appetite for satisfaction.

Decades ago, as I was sitting on the floor at my coffee table watching *Monday Night Football* and eating ice cream out of the carton, God suddenly blasted me with this truth: "There is not enough ice cream *in the world* to satisfy what you are trying to satisfy with it right now." I immediately put the spoon down, put what was left of the ice cream back in the freezer, and stood there feeling stunned. *Of course!* I thought to myself. *Duh! No wonder I eat until I'm more than full, and it still isn't enough!*

That was a turning point in my life as God really hammered home that point to me at almost every turn for quite a while after that. Back then, my propensity to overeat was almost a constant, and the Holy Spirit kept reminding me, "It's never enough." I look back now and can see how it was never enough and that it was *never* going to be enough because I was feeding an unholy urge to satisfy my sin nature.

Let me say that again. *I was feeding an unholy urge to satisfy my sin nature.* Heinous, indeed! It was like a fire that burned in me, and the more I fed it, the hotter it burned. One of my responses to this realization was that I developed some fairly strong beliefs and convictions about food and what *real* food is. Some of these beliefs may be only opinions, and some are truly just a fact, but I also believe that it is definitely an individual matter when it comes to determining what we think qualifies as good, bad, and ugly food.

## Sexy Food

What?! Food is *sexy*? Well, one definition of the word is "excitingly appealing." *Glamorous* would be another word you could use, which means to be charming or fascinatingly attractive. Junk food is sexy food in the sense that it is very tempting. Isn't that the way junk foods are put forth in commercials and how they are packaged and appear on store shelves? They are colorful and have exciting packaging and seductive advertising.

It's weird though. Shouldn't it be the drab, unattractive foods we *aren't* tempted by that companies ought to entice us to eat? I mean, did you ever notice nobody makes commercials about how irresistible their carrots are or how tempting their broccoli is? And surely none of us sits down to *Monday Night Football* with a crate full of apples or a pound of raw green beans where we have to resist eating all of them. No, we are only enticed by foods you might call seductive. They have to be "sexy" enough to get our attention and cause us to want to indulge, which usually results in *over*indulgence.

Consider those round, candy-coated chocolates. In one commercial, you'll see a sexy female candy talking in a smoky smooth voice to a male candy who comes across as kind of dopey. The packaging for these candies has happy, smiling faces that fairly say, "Eat me!" Or take those chocolate cake rolls in the snack food section with colorful, exciting graphics and enticing bigger-than-life pictures of the cake rolls that show the creamy goodness inside. If you look long enough, you've already started eating those scrumptious little cake rolls in your mind, which is just the effect the packaging is supposed to have. And then you *have* to buy them because you can't imagine getting home without them and not being able to finish the one you started "eating" in the store.

TV commercials have an even greater level of temptation because they use animation. I've noticed that breakfast cereal manufacturers have very creative commercials that can really affect your emotions, although what I am about to tell you is somewhat disturbing.

You've probably seen the commercial for a square, cinnamon-flavored breakfast cereal that depicts two squares standing next to each other. One of them furtively licks the other like it isn't supposed to notice getting licked. Another ad shows one square eating another one and declaring something like, "It must be all of that crunchy cinnamon goodness." Well, it's really creepy because what we're seeing is breakfast food cannibalism. Even worse is the ad where the cinnamon square eats *itself*. Anyway, I don't know how that is supposed to make you want to eat them, but it goes to show the lengths companies will go to charm you into eating.

And speaking of charms, one breakfast cereal has little marshmallow bits in it called "charms," and the cereal is called "lucky." How fun! Let's eat! See how it works? They put it forth like it's the pot of gold at the end of the rainbow, and they even have a leprechaun to show you the way! Rather, those marshmallow "charms" are more like death bombs for your body, and more than likely, it's children's bodies that have to endure them. I think you get the point. In fact, it tires me out to even write about this because we all know this already.

## Where Do We Draw the Line?

Let me just synopsize the chapter so far. Food exists to fuel our bodies, but there is a wide range of food, from whole foods to junk food. And as a society, we eat too little whole food and too much junk food, which we are easily tempted to do because of its appeal. The juncture we are at now is this: Where is the line between too much and too little? Where, indeed, do we draw the line?

At the beginning of Chapter 7, I talked about the lines we draw and should not cross in regard to our physical and mental capacities, like staying up too late, exercising too much, looking at a computer screen too long, or spending too many hours in a row trying to write a book! Man, sometimes I just can't even think anymore and know it's time to go pick up my guitar. Anyway, the point is that we only have so much energy, and we must respect the limits we have and live according to them.

It's different for each of us, so we must recognize that we are unique individuals with no two of us alike. There is no "one size fits all" when it comes to our physical limits. In the same way, we are individuals in regard to food, and most of us have probably spent a lot of our lives "drawing the line" in some way when it comes to food. But the question is this: Have we set the right limits and for the right reasons?

We know our own convictions about food and have consciences that tell us what is good, bad, or ugly and how much is too much or not enough. I can't really help you with that. What I can say is that you've got to follow what your conscience is telling you. Hopefully, if you are a believer in Jesus, your conscience won't be merely what you are saying to yourself but what the indwelling Holy Spirit is prompting and directing you to do. We'll get into that aspect in the next chapter, but for now....

## This is Really Good! Here, Try It!

Have you ever been at a meal with people, and when the dessert is served, the person next to you, being finicky and never having had the dessert before, waits until you try it? Then they ask, "Do you like it? Is it good?" They don't want to eat something that isn't good, so they want to be assured that they will like it. But there is a lot of room for opinion when it comes to food, so actually it's kind of useless to even ask. The point is that we don't want to experience something we don't like. We only want what is good, and when we've had it, we tend to recommend it to others.

So, here's my recommendation. Do what makes you happiest! Whoa! Do I really mean that? Maybe that makes you feel like all the rules are off, like it's a free-for all and you can eat to your heart's content! Well, you may be surprised to know that is exactly what I mean! But the real deal is, as we saw in the beginning chapters of this book, that you can't truly be happy unless you are holy. And holiness never includes gluttony or undisciplined living. True happiness only comes when we are obeying God, listening to the Holy Spirit's prompting, and doing what our consciences are telling us to do.

As you know, I have run the gamut from eating whatever I wanted whenever I wanted and overindulging in sugary foods to now only eating whole foods, including a lot of fresh greens, whole meats, fish, cheeses, nuts, and pre- and probiotic foods that support a healthy gut biome. I have never been more at peace, more in control of how I eat, or more satisfied with what I eat than I am today. And you know, I guess I can truly say that I eat whatever I want whenever I want it!

What makes that possible and so easy is that I truly don't want junk food anymore. I want to feed my body with only what is best for me, and there are a couple reasons for that. One is that I want to be as healthy and functional as possible. But the second and far more important reason is that I want to honor and glorify God. As we have seen, our bodies are the temple of the Holy Spirit, and how we care for our bodies and feed them is evidence of how much we honor and respect them (we talked about this in Chapter 7). This is a glorious place to be in, but the journey has been long and difficult. It's miraculous really, considering who I was and where I came from, but praise be to God that the way I eat now has made me happier and more content than I have ever been in my life. If that seems like an impossible dream to you, it was to me too. But nothing is impossible with God, so keep seeking Him and trusting Him to bring about miraculous changes in you.

## So, Here's My Opinion....

I don't eat anything I consider "bad" or "ugly" food, mainly because of what I think it is from a sort of spiritual point of view. So, what constitutes bad or ugly food? Let me just define ugly food. It has nearly zero nutritional value and is designed purely for our emotional enjoyment. It feeds our hearts and minds but not our bodies. And surely our bodies, if they could tell us, would say they don't enjoy ugly food and don't give them any more of it! Take gummy bears, for instance. They're made of glucose syrup, sugar, gelatin, flavoring, white and yellow beeswax, and food coloring. They're basically nutrition-free carbohydrates. *They're not food*! They're really not even made from stuff that was food to start with except for the glucose syrup that came from wheat or corn. But still, it left behind all its food value and only brought with it its ability to make you diabetic and fat.

So look, I'm not going to candy-coat what I have to say, but I might as well just say it. Ugly foods—mainly what we call junk food, cookies, candy bars, donuts, and even white flour, pasta, and bagels—are an adulteration of real food. People have taken the good stuff, whole foods, that God created and have corrupted them into flavors, colors, and textures to feed our emotions. These adulterations do harm to our bodies and do little to nothing to actually *feed* them. It's unholy stuff, I say!

All this junk works right into the devil's plan to tempt us away from what is good and get us addicted to what is bad for us. It's no wonder that we call ugly food "guilty pleasures" and "sinful delights" because they are!

Now, I'm not saying that everybody feels guilty when they eat junk like this, or that they *should* feel guilty, or even that they shouldn't eat stuff like this. I say it just to give a perspective. In my opinion, we are way better off never eating this junk because it really is poisonous, not only to our bodies but also to our hearts and souls.

The capacity for junk food to corrupt us is plain to see, and we have experienced this way too much for way too long. But for some of us, we can eat sugary treats without overindulging, without experiencing any temptation, and seeming to not suffer any ill effects physically. I say "seeming" because our bodies *do* suffer from junk food every time we eat it. And in proportion to the amount we eat, it just takes decades to blossom into diabetes. So that's my take, like it or not. All I can say is to listen to God the Holy Spirit within you and obey the promptings that He brings about in your conscience.

CHAPTER 10

# Our Goals, Our Weakness, and Our Power

Maybe by now you are convinced for the first time or the thousandth time that you need to make some changes in your relationship with food. And maybe you feel a bit more hopeful that it can happen, but a regretful history leaves a bad taste in your mouth.

Speaking of bad tastes, when you don't like the taste of something you eat, you generally don't eat it again. I mean, I'll never eat mango flavored frosting again, not only because I don't eat sugar but because when I did have some mango frosting, it tasted really bad. If you have the same opinion, we need not describe what it tasted like. Obviously, you won't eat it again, which makes sense. But why isn't it that simple with what we *do*?

Like, why do we do stuff over and over when we don't like the results of it? Most of us have probably done the "lose weight, gain weight" thing more than we want to remember, but why do we do that? For the simple reason that it tastes good! Well, not the whole process, losing weight doesn't taste nearly as good as when we are gaining it back. If only we disliked it as much as mango frosting, we'd be all set!

## We Need a Plan!

Most of us have been through this over and over, and we need a new path, a new "how to." Well, there isn't one, sorry. All we have is the same old tired plan: obey God. Now hold on! Don't throw up your hands and say, "That's easy for you to say" because, well, it *is* easy to say, but to *do* it? It's impossible. Only God Himself can bring about obedience in us, and that is what this chapter is all about.

Now, you may recall that I wrote at the beginning of Chapter 1:

> On the other hand, I really dislike Christian self-help books—the ones that say, "Ten steps to bliss in the Christian life." They are very light on theology or actually get it wrong. Many of them make *people* the focus and not God, which will not help anyone. But sometimes the format is helpful because taking certain steps in a certain order is necessary to accomplish something.

So, this surely is *not* a self-help book but definitely a God-help-me book, and what follows will not be "three steps to obeying God" but rather a discussion about what is really going on in our hearts, minds, and souls from a theological and psychological point of view.

As an example, my sister and I frequent a nice little diner down by the lake. The waitresses are classic diner waitresses—very friendly, attentive, and talkative. Two of them are trying to lose weight by cutting carbohydrate intake, basically doing keto. One of them talked about her travails with it each time we were there, about everything she "couldn't have." It really painted a bleak picture. My sis tried to tell her she ought to focus on what she *could* have, but it fell on deaf ears. The last time we were there, the waitress said nothing about the "diet." I think she doesn't have a problem with it anymore because she quit doing it. I'll ask her about it next time, but the point is that she bombed her efforts by focusing on the wrong thing. She only saw herself as deprived, and her whole demeanor was one of white-knuckling it until she made it through to her goal.

That kind of tension-producing mindset is just one of the many ways we can sabotage our efforts. But there are many more ways to doom our progress, so read on!

## Endgame

Action movies are cool because they have heroes who usually manage to bring about justice on the big bad guy who, in the end, gets what's coming to him. A recent movie based on a comic book series portrays just that, only there is a whole squad of superheroes trying to kill an epic bad guy who wants to rule the world. The heroes' goal is without debate—eliminate the bad guy and bring lasting peace to the world. They give all they have, one of them even his own life, to accomplish this. They didn't deviate, procrastinate, or rationalize but went after the bad guy with all haste. They had right motives, the right goal, and the power to do it. There are a lot of good lessons in this, the most important one being that their endgame was clear. They had no doubt about their goal and would accept nothing less than accomplishing it. After all, the fate of the world depended on it! Thankfully, we don't bear the same burden with our goals, but we must be similarly committed and clear on what our goals are.

## We Have Arrived…

To start with, we must know where we want to end, but the end isn't where you may think. This is not a race, nor a marathon, and it doesn't even have a finish line. Nor is it a place or a certain condition. But it is a *state of being*. And guess what? We have already arrived!

"What?" you may ask. "What do you mean?"

Well, for one thing, believing that you have already successfully finished before you even begin can be quite motivating and encouraging. Now, I'm not talking about the goals we have for our physical condition but about the most important aspect of ourselves, our soul, and our relationship with God. As believers in Jesus, we have "arrived" in a certain sense because we have been justified, are being sanctified, and will be glorified in the eternal state. But from God's perspective, it's all a done deal.

> *And these whom He predestined, He also called; and these whom He called, He also justified; and these whom He justified, He also glorified.*
> —Romans 8:30

Notice that "glorified" is in the past tense. Our destiny to be made perfect and live in the presence of God is assured, like it already *is*! It is a glorious future and ought to cause us to say, "How much more matters of this life?"

Another thing to keep in mind is that God has declared us to be holy and has given us the righteousness of Christ so He can say that we are His beloved children in whom He is well-pleased. That doesn't mean we always please Him, but He loves us and approves of us like the dearest, best dad you can imagine. I guess my point is that being loved like this and having the eternal destiny that we do ought to cause us to care far less about the present appearance and condition of our physical bodies while at the same time giving us the motivation to take good care of them. And a good, right motivation is what we need.

## But When Do We Get There?

Goals are important, but they can also sabotage our efforts. When we say we want to lose 20 pounds and finally do it, whew! We made it! Then what happens after that? First, we rejoice, and then we ease off on restrictions or throw them off completely and immediately begin to regress. Once we go backward far enough and get upset with what we look like, we'll kick on the diet again.

The whole problem with this is that our goal was wrong, and it was wrong in two ways. First of all, we made it mostly about what we *look like*. And that actually causes the second problem—we get into a mental race or journey to get to that mile marker that says we have lost 20 pounds. As I have said, goals are important, but wrong goals will cause problems with the efforts we are making to get there and likely prevent us from accomplishing them at all.

Another problem is that our emotional state can be negatively affected when our current weight isn't what we think it should be or want it to be. That can cause us to become even more focused on our appearance and alter how we feel toward ourselves. As you know, I suffered a lot growing up with shame for being fat, and as long as we still think we are fat, we are likely to continue the process of shaming ourselves until we arrive at that mile post. The urgency to get there can sometimes be overwhelming since we have so closely tied our "self" to our body condition. And if you're a black-and-white, all-or-nothing kind of person, that can have us condemning ourselves nearly to hell until we get the weight off. Or if we lose the 20 pounds, we can tend to raise ourselves to almost angelic status and feel ecstatic about ourselves. Surely, we must not let our body condition so affect our mental and emotional state!

A third problem with specific weight loss goals is that life goes on after we get there! I know from personal experience that we are not usually prepared for that. Our whole focus has been on the 20 pounds or a certain look, and when we finally see the right numbers on the scale or the right look in the mirror, we then look ahead and have no plan on how to reach the next marker.

Certainly, if we have just lost 20 pounds and that was our goal, something has to change with how we are eating and exercising, or we will keep losing weight. Obviously, we have to eat more, and since "diets" require rather spartan amounts and unsatisfying kinds of foods, we naturally will go for the foods that will have us gaining what we just lost. This whole process of measuring ourselves by the pound tends to not only cause our weight to go up and down but our emotions to go for a ride, too, and that is not good for us at all. Thankfully, the solution to this *is* good for us.

## We Never Get There

Automobiles are not alive (obvious, I know), although some people give them names and love them like they are. I named my car and the two previous ones I had. Someone I know had a Ford Explorer and named it Dora. There's nothing wrong with this, but it shows that we have certain sentiments toward our cars. Some of us care very much what they look like and how clean they are, while others never wash them and don't care a lick about the rust and dented bumpers. But one thing we all have in common is that we care whether our vehicles function correctly. We have them for a purpose—to take us places. No one would put their money into making the car look good when they need to spend it on getting it to run.

Similarly, our physical body is a tool. It carries our souls around and enables us to perceive and experience the material world. And I think that we all care that it functions correctly. This ought to be our goal, to be as fit and functional as God calls and enables each one of us to be.

I want to emphasize the "each one of us" part. As unique individuals, we each have our own capacities, beliefs, and desires in regard to our physical condition or fitness. Some don't care if they are rusty and dented, while others want to be all glossy and smooth. Either way is fine. There is nothing wrong with wanting our bodies to look a certain way or not caring what they look like at all, but what we look like can't be our motivation for getting fit and optimally functional. Our primary goal must be fitness.

All our eating and exercising must have as its prime objective to make us healthy and fit. If we go for appearance first, we *will* fail. Even if we do manage to get ourselves to look the way we want to, the tendency toward pride about it and self-exaltation can be high. If we engage in that, then that is where the failure happens.

So then what? Do you ever get to look how you want to? Maybe. But the good thing is that for those of us who want to look good, to *look* physically fit, we usually will once we *are* fit.

## *The Pursuit of Fitness*

There was a really good book published in the late 1970s called *The Pursuit of Holiness*. And surprise! It was all about being holy! As we talked about in Chapter 3, we must seek to be holy in all our thoughts and actions. That takes discipline and effort, which God commands and enables, so we progress in holiness, becoming incrementally more like Jesus.

Holiness is the highest spiritual ideal we must strive after, and it is somewhat like a fitness of the soul. It is being "fitted" or suited for the specific purpose of worshiping God. The more holy we are, the more able we are to perceive and experience God. That results in loving Him more and more, and that love naturally glorifies Him as we rejoice in Him. But as we know, the pursuit of holiness is lifelong and will end only when we see Jesus face to face. Oh, what a day that will be! For now, we pursue holiness with our spiritual eyes on Him.

So ought our pursuit of physical fitness be. It's a day-by-day, lifelong pursuit. Just as we engage every day in the spiritual disciplines of Bible reading, studying, memorizing, and prayer, we must engage in physical disciplines such as walking, running, weight training, bicycling, swimming, and eating good whole foods. As I said, this must be a lifelong effort, and as you persist in it and time passes, your body *will* change. Your musculature will tone up and your body fat will decrease.

It's inevitable as long as you are diligent in it. And let me say that the longer you keep at it and practice good habits, the easier and more comfortable it gets. Someday you may even come to the place where you ask yourself, "How could I ever have chosen to live any other way?" I certainly did, and it is more than worth the initial sacrifices I had to make. I look back and can say that they were not really sacrifices at all, considering what I gained by them.

## *A Quick Tip*

I'm not a nutritionist, dietician, nor am I approved by the FDA, but I know a bit about how our bodies function and have learned it the hard way. After decades of failure at losing body fat and having believed the conventional wisdom that dietary fat is bad for you, that low calories are a must, and all other kinds of baloney, I found that it comes down to a really simple principal. When you eat fatty, high-carb foods, your body burns some of the carbs and stores the fat. If you eat low-fat, high-carb foods, you will burn some and store the rest as fat.

Because these kinds of foods make up most of the standard American diet, our bodies are trained to burn carbohydrates for energy. They don't really know how to burn fat for energy because there are usually so many carbs available. If you reduce carb intake, especially processed carbs like bread and pasta, your body will have to use fat for energy, and over the long haul, it will gradually adapt to that.

A good rule of thumb for meals is moderate protein, high fat, and low carbs (15 grams or less) *or* moderate protein, low fat (5 grams), and high carbs (not more than 50 grams). Only very rarely should you eat meals with equal amounts of carbs and fat because we automatically store the fat when carbs are present. It's simple and scientifically sound! For more information on how our bodies burn fat, look up how insulin levels affect fat loss. That is really the key.

## Our Weakness

We're full of it! Weakness that is, and hopefully, according to past failures, we can agree with this. My mom's neighbor had this amazing hedgerow. He trimmed it to be square, and it went from the front of his house up to the road. As the years went by, it got taller and taller, and eventually, he fashioned an arched doorway in it. It looked pretty cool. He was fastidious about trimming it and did so every couple of weeks. For some reason, though, he left the trimmings on my mom's side of the yard, and they lay there in the grass, going from green to wilted to brown in just a couple days. Eventually they got mowed and mulched by her lawnmower....

Jesus said in John 15:5, "I am the vine, you are the branches; he who abides in Me and I in him, he bears much fruit, for apart from Me you can do nothing." Without Jesus, we can do *nothing*. We have as much ability as those dry, dead trimmings had to jump up and graft themselves back into the hedge and be a living, productive part of the plant. Simply put, we're all weakness and no power! If you're not convinced yet, read on, and hopefully we will all have a more accurate belief of our weakness and a greater understanding of...

## The Power of God

This is a big topic. I mean big, *really* big, like there literally is nothing bigger. God's power is as infinite as He is. Everything about God is infinite—His love, grace, and mercy have no end. We can't fully comprehend infinite things, but we understand the concept. So, what is God's power, and how is it available to us?

These are necessary questions to answer since we are powerless and need His power if we are to accomplish anything. To begin with, God's power *creates*. And He creates stuff out of nothing. Who else can do that? When He said, "Let there be light," light appeared. And so it was with everything that exists. He made it all and, man alive, there is *a lot* of it! Not only the sheer mass of it but also the microscopic complexity of it.

### *Space, the Final Frontier*

One sci-fi TV show said that space was the final frontier, but I think what is beyond space is the final frontier, the place we all want to be with God Himself. But even the size of space is unbelievable. Scientists measure distance in space by how far light travels in one year, and they call that unit a light year. Since light travels at 186,000 miles per second, it's not surprising that it travels almost 6 trillion miles in a year. That is an incomprehensible distance, but what is worse is trying to comprehend the distance across our Milky Way galaxy. It is 180,000 light years from end to end. Multiply 180,000 times 6 trillion, and that's how many miles it is across our little galaxy. But there are 100 billion to 200 billion *more* galaxies! And to think that God is bigger than all of that and exists outside of it … like, does He *encompass* all those trillions of trillions of miles of space and matter?

*Weather or Not....*
Or consider the power of weather such as hurricanes or tornadoes. A lightning bolt has 300 million volts in it compared to 120 volts in household current. And we have all seen or experienced the devastating power of a hurricane and the terrible and uncontrollable forces of storm surges and flooding that come with it. Tornadoes lift cars into the air and tear whole buildings off their foundations.

The power we see in weather is hard to quantify but imagine that a single dollar bill represented the total power of every hurricane, lightning bolt, and tornado that has ever occurred. How would God's power compare to that? Picture bundles of $100 bills stacked six feet high filling your whole living room. That's maybe $1.5 billion.

Of course, God's power is infinite, so we would need more living rooms than just yours. Indeed, we would need whole planets of living rooms and beyond that a bunch more galaxies. But even the estimated 150 billion galaxies that exist wouldn't have enough living rooms full of money to compare God's power to the dollar bill worth of power we have experienced with weather on this planet. It's incomprehensible, really. The power we see in nature is indeed awesome and fearful, but it is nothing compared to God's power.

## *The Knowledge of God*

DNA … deoxyribonucleic … Dang! I almost spelled it right, but the wavy red line showed me otherwise. Spell check to the rescue! At least I sort of know what DNA is.

As I have maybe made clear by now, I didn't become very educated in high school, but I can look stuff up on the old interwebs, and so I am! Consider our DNA. It's the stuff that contains our genetic information. Like an instruction manual, DNA is double helix structures coiled up within the cells of our bodies that instruct the cells on how to behave or what to produce.

Now, there is a lot of complexity to that whole process, which I am going to skip because this isn't science class, and I certainly don't know enough to write about it. I want to get to the part about how much genetic information is contained in each of our bodies.

So, the science isn't exact on how many cells are in our bodies, but estimates are about 30 trillion. The double helix ladder of DNA is coiled up to fit in each cell, but if it is uncoiled and stretched out, it is 6 feet long! From a single cell! The "letters" of information on this strand are microscopic, so there are a *whole bunch* of them in 6 feet of space. Multiply that 6 feet times the number of cells in our bodies, and we get 3.4 billion miles of information!

And while most of this information is the same for each of us, there are slight variations and mutations, but God knows *all* of this. He could tell us, cell by cell, how the 7.7 billion people in this world are different from each other, down to every individual cell! My mind is boggled just looking at the grass in my yard and thinking that God knows how many blades there are….

The absolute, comprehensive knowledge that God has of every single thing that exists is indeed mind-blowing. And not only does He *know* it, but He thought it all up and *created* it! And He sovereignly *controls* all of it!

## The Fuse Is Blown!

Yeah, maybe our mind fuse is blown trying to comprehend the knowledge and power of God, but I'm talking about fuses in a fuse box. We've all experienced it. We're innocently sitting at our computer or by a lamp reading a book, and *blamo!* The power goes out. You go out of the room and see that the power is still on in other parts of the house, but the microwave your teenager was using is off, as is the coffee pot and the new electric heater your spouse was trying out, all on the same circuit your reading room is on. Thankfully, getting the power going again is a simple matter of replacing the fuse.

But sometimes the power is out in the whole house, and it's not just the fuses. You look out into the neighborhood, and everything is dark with not a light to be seen. What do we do then? Call the power company and find out what has happened and when we can expect the power to come back on. In the meantime (generators aside), we are helpless to do anything but wait. Maybe we can light a candle and read a book, but otherwise we are almost wholly dependent on electricity to be able to do anything in our houses.

Thus it is with the power we need to accomplish anything in our lives. We must wait upon the Lord and look to Him to empower us.

## Loose Connections

One day I was sitting in my music-drawing-writing room, and I thought I smelled something hot, like electrical hot. I went to the laundry room, and as I got closer to the fuse box, the smell got stronger. Putting my hand on the cover of the fuse box, I found that it was warm. I called my husband (the cover is getting warmer and the burning smell stronger), and he asks if I have been running the small electric heater in my room. I said yes, and he asked where I have it plugged in. When I tell him, he says to turn it off. So I do, and the heat and smell dissipate.

I open the fuse box door and see a wire that is somewhat melted and determine that it is not screwed down tight. The problem was that electric heaters draw a lot of current, and the loose screw was impeding the flow of the current, causing it to overheat. I don't know how the screw got loose (I think maybe the way the washing machine would sometimes rumble on the spin cycle), but obviously loose connections are very dangerous in fuse boxes.

But loose connections are also dangerous in a spiritual sense. We need to be tight with God. Our connection needs to be solid if we are going to have the power to do what He wants us to do. If our connection to Him is loose, we will "overheat" and ultimately fail. We've all felt it. We try so hard to accomplish something, but eventually we flame out. At least the overheating of failure doesn't actually light us on fire, but if it did, it might wake us up to how much we need God.

## How Do We Plug In?

How many times have we struggled to get something to work, and someone comes up and says, "Well, is it plugged in?" You scowl and glare, but as the person picks up the unplugged cord, your face changes quite a bit. Things that are powered by electricity need to be plugged into a source of electricity if they are to function (another obvious statement, I know).

So how do we "plug in" to the power of God? I put "plug in" in quotes because technically we *already are* connected to the power of God, or more accurately, we already *possess* the power of God. And really, it's not a possessing but a *presence* since the Holy Spirit dwells within us.

I am tempted to go into a deep theological exposition of the Holy Spirit's role in our lives, but there are probably books about that, so I'll keep it short and sweet. The main thing is that as the Holy Spirit resides within us, He is the source of power and actuating force in our lives, enabling us to do everything God commands us to do.

> *Do you not know that you are a temple of God and that the Spirit of God dwells in you?*
> —1 Corinthians 3:16

What does "dwell" mean? Simply put, it means to reside in a house, to occupy, and by implication, to co-habit. So, the Holy Spirit lives in us and inhabits every part of our being. His presence is the power of God within us.

> *For it is God who is at work in you, both to will and to work for His good pleasure.*
> —Philippians 2:13

God is our power, but the following shows how we have our part to play:

> *For this purpose also I labor, striving according to His power, which mightily works within me.*
> —Colossians 1:29

We have to labor or make the effort to accomplish what is before us to do, but God is our power in doing it. So, if the very power of Almighty God is in us and available for us to accomplish all His will, why do we so often fail?

## Throw the Switch!

You know how in movies there will be some big, dramatic thing going on, and they *have* to get the power on in the building so the computers work, and they can save the world? Time is running out, but eventually a few of them get to the basement, looking frantically with their flashlights, and find the circuit board. The big H-shaped main power handle switch thingie is in the off position, and one of them dives for it and flips it up. The power comes on, the computers light up, the signal goes out, and the world is saved!

Well, that's not how it works with the power of God in us. If only we *could* flip a switch and have God empowering us all the time at full power. Unfortunately, we short-circuit His work in us in many different ways.

## *Disobedience*

When we disobey God in some area of our lives, it affects all the other areas. That is because we are *one* soul. Contrary to popular characterization, we don't have compartments that make parts of ourselves separate and unaffected by the others. We're like a swimming pool—one big space.

Okay, so I don't like dogs much, and I've never been anywhere that the dog has been in the swimming pool. But if I were and if he had been, I sure wouldn't go swimming. Why? Because if the dog peed in the pool, well, it's everywhere! There's nowhere that the water is uncontaminated.

Sin affects us similarly. It indeed gets everywhere, and I believe it inhibits the power of the Spirit in us. First Thessalonians 5:19 commands us, "Do not quench the Spirit," but that's what we do when we willfully sin. If we are to succeed in what God has called us to do, we must be engaged in it with a whole heart. No sinning with anything anywhere!

## *Laziness*

Nobody wants to be lazy, but it's what our sin nature wants, so we have to fight against it. The easy way out never gets you anywhere that you want to be. In fact, you'll never get anywhere because the way of the lazy is like a hedge of thorns (Prov. 15:19). I've tried getting through a regular hedge, and thick, interwoven branches made it impossible. Imagine one with thorns. Doing the hard work of sawing and chopping is the only way through, so let us follow Paul's example.

*But by the grace of God I am what I am, and His grace toward me did not prove vain; but I labored even more than all of them, yet not I, but the grace of God with me.*
—1 Corinthians 15:10

Paul worked hard. And he was diligent. He labored. He stuck to it and saw it through no matter what it took. We must do the same. Laziness short-circuits God's power in us because He can't empower an action that we are not taking. Now, this might sound like we have to take an action before He can empower it, but actually we are impelled to take action by God, and by His power we begin it and then carry it out. It's like when Jesus raised Lazarus from the dead. Jesus commanded, and Lazarus obeyed. Lazarus didn't raise himself, and yet it was he who got up and walked out of the tomb.

*Self-Effort*
Self-effort is where we try really hard, make up mottoes or slogans, visualize success, and vow to keep on until we make it. I unwittingly tried this for years and years. Fail every time!

Some call this kind of trying "willpower," but consider the word itself: "will" = "decision" and "power" = "ability." So "decision" + "ability" = success! That formula works, and even though I'm not good at math, I can see that for us puny, weak humans, we're missing half of the equation.

We don't have any power or ability at all. We must not foolishly assume that when we put "will" together with "power" we then have the power to carry out the thing we willed. To believe this is a major problem, so let's dig into it.

## The Myth of Willpower

Wanting to do something and *willing* to do it are two different things. So, we must be careful not to confuse "will" with "want to." If wanting to was all it took, we would all have achieved our dreams by now, but accomplishing anything significant requires an "I will." To say that we *will* do something is to say that we have made a definite decision. Inherent in such a positive declaration is a unity of purpose, an agreement with ourselves that we *will do* what we have stated we will do. This decision doesn't really take any effort since all it took was thinking. But to begin to actually *do* the thing and stick with it, that's where the effort comes in. Our "will" must *take action*!

Now, in our day-to-day lives, we "will" all kinds of things and do them without a second thought, like "I will stop at the store on the way home," or "I will work on writing my book," or "I will cook dinner now." But we never even think about willpower in these activities because they really take very little effort. Really, we just make a decision and then do it.

It is only when something is difficult that we think we need willpower. And when we fail, we wrongly assume that we didn't try hard enough, so we take a big breath and try harder. But it wasn't a lack of effort or power at all that caused the failure; it was our will that changed. See, it's not about how hard we try but rather that we *agree* with ourselves about what we *will* do. When we decide on a course of action and are 100 percent in agreement with it, it's smooth sailing! No willpower is necessary.

The problem comes, though, when it starts to feel difficult. It's not *really* more difficult, but it only *feels* that way. And that feeling of difficulty comes because our will *begins to waver*. We start to question whether it is worth the effort or the sacrifice. There are some chinks in the armor of our initial decision, and if we don't recommit and reaffirm, we will change our "will" to a "won't." Now, this questioning of our will doesn't usually happen quickly or plainly or simply. But there is a lot of subterfuge going on, brought about by the world, the devil, and our sinful bent toward comfort and ease. Any one of these factors can start to talk to us, to argue for a different course of action. And if we are unaware of or untrained to recognize this, we will quickly succumb and decide to alter our course from our original goal.

This is where we make up stories and tell ourselves that it was too difficult or that we don't want to anymore. But we really still want to, and it really isn't too difficult. Technically, we are still *able* to continue to do the thing we had decided to do, but it is our will that said, "I'm not going to do that anymore." Once we have made that decision, no amount of willpower can change it because willpower and our conscious, positive decision can't even get into the same ring to duke it out.

So-called willpower is useless against a self-proclaimed "I won't." It's futile, in fact, and like the sci-fi TV show where an alien species tries to assimilate other species. They drive up in their giant spaceship cube and declare, "You shall be assimilated. Resistance is futile." And so it goes with the hapless other aliens. They get assimilated and turned into drones in the giant alien collective. That's what happens with willpower when we say we won't do something anymore.

Resistance to your own decision is indeed futile. I mean, think about that, and let me repeat it. *Resistance to your own decision is indeed futile.* It's like we're telling ourselves yes and no at the same time. So, forget about willpower because it's *not real!* But what we are saying to ourselves *is* real. How we debate with ourselves and the conclusions we come to in these debates are what actually determines what we do. But do we even realize what we are saying or who we are saying it to? This is the crucial subject of the next section.

## Don't Turn Into Your Parents!

The good news is that you can't become your parents because ... you already *are*! And you're still the kid you were too!

What?!

This becomes apparent when we pay attention to the conversations that we are having within ourselves. Parents talk to children, and children talk to parents. Now, when kids are growing up, these conversations can be quite predictable. Mom says, "Put your toys away," and little Jimmy says, "No!" Mom says, "Stop that!" and Jimmy says, "No!" Mom: "Put that back!" Jimmy: "No!" The fight for supremacy rages, but the wise parent knows how to bring Jimmy into line and has the authority to do it.

None of us would find it very admirable if a little kid demanded cookies before dinner and mom said okay. Then he wants two pieces of cake for dessert, and she says, "I guess it's all right this one time." And then Jimmy wants to stay up past his bedtime to watch a special program on TV, and again, she agrees! Mom rationalizes that it's okay because the next day is Saturday (even though they have an early morning soccer game to be at).

No doubt you can see where I am going with this. *We treat ourselves the same way!* Our conversations with ourselves are quite similar. The "parent" in us lets the "child" in us do whatever we want to much of the time. For example, we decide to cut out sugary carbs for the day, but halfway through, our "child" starts to complain. They begin to set forth their case for why they should be allowed to have that pumpkin walnut muffin you bought earlier in the week. "Well, I *am* hungry. It only has a few more carbs than the banana. It might be stale later…." And the rationalizing goes on until the child in you wins.

See? Willpower has nothing to do with it. It's about the *decisions* we make. And as you can see, right when it seems most difficult to maintain our will, the parent in us is usually having a heated discussion with the child in us who is trying to change the will of the parent. When we give in and let the child have their way, that is where we fail. But it wasn't a lack of willpower; it was a choice. I mean, all you have to do is really notice the dialogue that you're having with yourself when you feel like you need willpower to stay the course.

But staying on course doesn't take willpower; it takes a choice. Your parent voice must tell the child what you *will* do. End of story. No willpower is needed. So, let's forget about willpower and trying harder and trust God to empower our will while we focus on being faithful to Him.

## That Kid Has a Mind of His Own

Kids who have a mind of their own are generally disobedient and out of control. They don't listen, and they don't respect authority. Their actions usually produce bad results. They also have parents who are not holding them to account and *requiring* their obedience. But we are hardly any different when it comes to doing what we have agreed that we will do.

These dialogues we have with ourselves or with the Holy Spirit, arguing for a way out of our decision, are really no different than a kid arguing with their mom. Sometimes these debates can seem insurmountable, though, and we wind up giving in to what the child in us is demanding. I mean, I've seen it at the grocery store. A little kid is sitting in the cart in the checkout line and wants a candy bar that he sees. He can't reach it, so he starts saying, "I want it." But then mom says no.... Well, it makes me want to get into a different line. The calls for the candy bar increase in intensity and duration until the mom gives in, just to get the child to be quiet.

Many times, we do the same thing with ourselves, and usually when the stakes are high. We argue for the candy bar, and if we are not aware of the forces at work, we will likely give in. And it's not because we didn't try hard enough. It's because we *decided* to.

Why would we? A number of pages ago, I said, "But there is a lot of subterfuge going on, brought about by the world, the devil, and our sinful bent toward comfort and ease." It is vital to see how these three things can impact how we feel and how they can subtly influence our decision-making.

## The World

We've kind of gone over this in the previous chapter—how "the world," as in our American culture, puts before our eyes all kinds of things that we just have to have or experience. It's like, "You deserve a break today," or "Have it your way." Or it's the allurements of a bacon cheddar cheeseburger where they show the cheese slowly melting and the scrumptious juices flowing. And it's usually in slow motion and close-up, which is not a lot different from the way lingerie is advertised. They make you want it, and the battle begins.

At least the battle had *better* begin or we will lose it before we even know it's there. We have to fight against the world's enticements. The "you've got to have this" advertising, especially when it comes to food, really plays on our bodily appetites.

## The Flesh

Our "flesh" is that sinful, irredeemable, God-hating part of us that always seeks to satisfy itself in unholy ways. It is a burning furnace stoked by what we see, hear, and believe. And if we take these truths lightly or are unaware of this, we will be ruled by it and fall victim to its attempts to subvert all our efforts to live in accord with God's will. Just like some young children, our bodies have a mind of their own, and we must, by God's power, rule over them.

The Apostle Paul said, "But I discipline my body and make it my slave, so that, after I have preached to others, I myself will not be disqualified" (1 Cor. 9:27). To *discipline* means to "bring into subjection" or "be a slave driver." We *must* deal with our sin nature so it's not driving us to temptation with such ferocity that we succumb to it.

## The Devil

Satan works in concert with the way the world tempts us and our sin nature to entice us *personally*. He knows your weaknesses. Recently a friend of mine was really struggling with eating too much frozen custard from a local retail location. Satan knew this and so didn't bother tempting her with pizza or apple pies. He knew the custard would be the hardest thing to resist, and he even knew the specific flavor, so he sent his minions with one directive: "Tempt her with the vanilla almond custard. Tell her she can't do without it." He knows how to get to us, and he will use everything at his disposal to do so.

## Keep Off the Grass!

Sometimes our struggle isn't even with the world's allurements, our sin nature's "mind of its own" or the devil's special temptations. It is just with the simple "you're not allowed to do that" kind of thing. When you're not supposed to do something, sometimes it gets to be all you think about. It's like the waitress I talked about at the beginning of this chapter. All she thought about on her diet was what she couldn't have, and it eventually drove her to just give in and quit the diet. She finally just walked on the grass and felt a huge relief. We must be very wary of this kind of "you're not allowed to" or "who are you to tell me what to do?" or "you can't make me."

## Did You Hear That?

Imagine that you're watching a scary movie, and there are two teenagers in the basement of a really old house. They've heard that the house is haunted, and they are nervous. But they are down there trying to find a box of old, vinyl records. The lights don't work, so they are using a flashlight. Suddenly there is a clunking sound, and one of them whispers, "Did you hear that?" They both freeze and listen very intently....

This is what we must do when it comes to hearing what we are saying to ourselves because sadly, some of us are not very well plugged in to our internal dialogue and will almost unknowingly rationalize and quit without even a chance of rebuttal. So, let's listen carefully to what is being said within us because our success in remaining true to ourselves and, more importantly, true to God is at stake. If those teenagers had been listening carefully in the first place, they would have realized that the clunking sound came from upstairs where the other kids were and therefore would have had a more appropriate response to it.

## "I Wonder, Is It Just Me or . . ."

There is another angle to this parent-child analogy, and it has to do with who we are talking to when we are trying to get out of a thing we have committed to do. I'm no psychologist (I can't even spell the word, and I got it so wrong that spell check didn't even have a suggestion), nor am I a theologian. Sometimes I feel like I'm just making stuff up, but I guess it's my experience, so here goes. Hopefully, you get what I mean by the dialogue we have with ourselves between "parent" and "child," so you can also understand a far more important point about who this "parent" and "child" can be sometimes.

I think usually we're just going back and forth with ourselves, but sometimes this "parent" can be the Holy Spirit speaking to us. It may be God Himself reminding us of our commitment and commanding us to stay the course. Conversely, no doubt you can see who the "child" is. Satan's whisperings and cajolings also speak to us to tempt us, turn us, discourage us, and get us to give up.

We *must* hear these things and, by God's grace and power, reject them and stand firm in our convictions. It's all part of keeping the faith. It goes back to the point I made in Chapter 8 about halfway through in the section called "Keeping the Covenant." When we decide to do a thing, like committing to eat a certain way, we are not only committing to ourselves to do it but more importantly, we are committing to God.

If we are indeed doing all to the glory of God as 1 Corinthians 10:31 commands, then anything and everything we do must be consecrated to Him. And maybe more compelling is the following:

> *Whatever you do in word or deed, do all in the name of the Lord Jesus, giving thanks through Him to God the Father.*
> —Colossians 3:17

I hope and pray that this provokes a deep conviction in you about how serious our decisions and "I wills" are. Not only must we do all to the glory of God, but it must be consecrated in Jesus' name. Surely this sheds new light on what it means to give in to the "child" within us who argues for his own way. How dare we, then, argue with the Holy Spirit and try to rationalize eating that pumpkin walnut muffin or worse, agree with the "child" when it may very well be Satan himself trying to get us to fold.

Now, I'm not saying that taking action in accord with a decision we made is easy or doesn't take effort but remember that it is God Himself by the indwelling Holy Spirit who will empower that effort in us. And we can be sure that He will if we are fighting to maintain our commitment to an action we have consecrated in Jesus' name to the glory of God. So keep watch, and really listen to what is going on in your heart and mind.

> *Therefore let him who thinks he stands take heed that he does not fall. No temptation has overtaken you but such as is common to man; and God is faithful, who will not allow you to be tempted beyond what you are able, but with the temptation will provide the way of escape also, so that you will be able to endure it.*
> —1 Corinthians 10:12–13

CHAPTER 11

# How We Function

So far, it could seem like this book has focused on why we eat, what we eat, and what we try not to eat so we can enjoy food however we like and look the way we want to. But obviously, it's been far more about *who we are*. It's been about what we believe, our perspective on things, how we each deal with difficult goals, and the mental, emotional, and spiritual aspect of ourselves.

This stuff matters *way more* than the condition of our bodies or what we look like. A favorite phrase of mine is this: "It doesn't matter what you look like; it's who you are that matters...." I left this open ended because there is a second half to it that I will get to in the next chapter. But for our immediate purposes, this statement can stand on its own.

## A Famous Theologian Once Said....

Well, I don't want to quote this theologian, or I'd have to go and get permission and all that, but he made the point that we aren't bodies with souls but souls with bodies. It is our *souls* that make us persons; it's where our identity and our character reside. It is our souls that are made in the image of God. It is our souls that think and feel and love. Our bodies are merely the vessels in which all this exists.

And we need our bodies because they are the physical means by which we operate in this material world. We need our physical brains to think, our ears to hear, our eyes to see, our vocal cords to speak, and so on. These are all means by which we receive and express information and feelings. So, our bodies are important, but only as a tool for the function of our souls. We are indeed souls with a body, and not the other way around.

## Overhaulin'

Ted had taken great pains with his old car, trying to make it look nice. It was a good old American muscle car, built to look good and go fast, and it had looked good. But now it was 40 years old, rusty, and tired. Ted had spent a lot of time smoothing out the dents and patching it up with Bondo, but it never looked how he wanted it to.

His geeky neighbor who drove an electric car that looked like a toaster used to chide him, saying, "Teddy! What's with all the useless effort on the car? It gets you to work every day, doesn't it?"

It was true; his car was very dependable because he kept up with maintenance, and it had never let him down. After more months of being teased, Ted began to think he really was wasting time and effort, so he let off on trying to make his car look better. That resulted in having more time and resources for more important things, like considering what sort of condition his heart and soul were in.

## Heart, Soul, and Mind

So, it doesn't matter what our bodies look like, and in some respects, it doesn't even matter how they function. This is because the proper functioning of our bodies is not necessary for our existence or relationship with God. We all have different levels of physical capabilities due to age, fitness, disease, or injury. But regardless of that, God has given us one ultimate command that we all can obey.

*And you shall love the Lord your God with all your heart, and with all your soul, and with all your mind, and with all your strength.*
—Mark 12:30

We obey this command with our *souls*, and that should tell us something about how important our bodies are—not very. But our souls are everything because our souls are our essence; they are *us*! So, the condition of our souls and our hearts and minds are what really matters. This is where *fitness* really matters. But we're so fixated on our bodies that we can't help but think of the word *physical* right before we say "fitness." Really, our souls need food, clothing, and shelter much more than our bodies do.

## *The Food of God*

We need food. Certainly, our bodies need food, and being deprived of it has fairly quick consequences. Too bad our souls don't complain as loudly when they get hungry because feeding them is far more important than feeding our bodies. And it's not enough just to keep our souls from being hungry. We ought to pack them with as much nutrition as possible—no spiritual gummy bears!

*Your words were found and I ate them, and Your words became for me a joy and the delight of my heart; for I have been called by Your name, O Lord God of hosts.*
—Jeremiah 15:16

If taking in God's word gives us joy and delight of heart, what happens if we don't ingest it? At the least, we'll have lack of joy and little delight. But generally, when we don't engage in the spiritual disciplines of reading, memorizing, and studying the Bible, we will be "eating" something else that is not as good for us and many times is actually damaging to us. Remember, too, that God says, "The joy of the Lord is your strength" (Neh. 8:10).

Jesus is the Word of God and the bread of life. "He who eats this bread will live forever" (John 6:58). The intake of God's word is critical to the health of our souls. It feeds us and strengthens us, brings health to us, and grants us joy. Our souls *need* God's word!

> *My son, give attention to my words; incline your ear to my sayings. Do not let them depart from your sight; keep them in the midst of your heart. For they are life to those who find them and health to all their body. Watch over your heart with all diligence, for from it* flow *the springs of life.*
> —Proverbs 4:20–23

## The Clothing of God

This world is a hostile environment to our hearts and minds, so we must be protected from it. Imagine being outside without a coat or shoes when it is below freezing. Or how about standing on burning sand with bare feet and the sun beating down on bare skin? You're either frozen or burned to a crisp! So, we protect ourselves from either of those fates by being properly clothed, but our spiritual protection and health are far more important than that.

> *But put on the Lord Jesus Christ, and make no provision for the flesh in regard to* its *lusts.*
> —Romans 13:14

> *Put on the full armor of God, so that you will be able to stand firm against the schemes of the devil.*
> —Ephesians 6:11

> *But since we are of* the *day, let us be sober, having put on the breastplate of faith and love, and as a helmet, the hope of salvation.*
> —1 Thessalonians 5:8

*So, as those who have been chosen of God, holy and beloved, put on a heart of compassion, kindness, humility, gentleness and patience; bearing with one another, and forgiving each other, whoever has a complaint against anyone; just as the Lord forgave you, so also should you. Beyond all these things* put on *love, which is the perfect bond of unity.*
—Colossians 3:12–14

That's a lot to put on! But we must be so clothed if our souls are to be healthy and fit. So get into the Word, obey the Word, and get your soul properly clothed!

## *The Shelter of God*

This isn't as easy to describe, but it is similar to how clothing shelters our bodies. I think being sheltered in God is not only to be protected by Him—well, wait. Imagine this. You're in the middle of nowhere, in a blinding snowstorm, your car quits running, your phone is dead. And just as you're starting to get cold, there's a knock on your window. It's some bearded guy in a winter parka with a pack and snowshoes on. He can't help you with the car, but he straps his extra pair of snowshoes on you and helps you trek to his house, miles away. Once you're inside, he gets a fire going, and you sit near it to warm up.

So, God has saved us from death and is our shelter. Indeed, scripture defines Him as our fortress, our strong tower, and our shield, and that under His wings we seek refuge. But there is another important aspect to God being our shelter. Once saved from the storm, we're going to want to talk to the guy who saved us, to thank him, and to get to know him and listen to him. Not only because we are grateful for being saved but also because we need his directions to get to the town where we can find a tow truck.

When we find our shelter in God, we must also find fellowship with Him. Our souls need Him like this. So, it is paramount for the health of our souls that we feed, clothe, and shelter ourselves in God through His word. That is what makes us *who we are*. I mean, think of it. For those who have died and are in the presence of God, they don't have bodies, but they are still just as much themselves, just as much who they are without bodies. Their essence, character, and personality are still intact—no bodies necessary!

## We Need Our Bodies

With all this talk of how irrelevant our bodies are, in a certain sense, we really do need them to live in this world. As we have seen, we can obey God's ultimate commandment without bodies. However, God's second command is to love our neighbor as ourselves, which does, in most instances, require a body. It's kind of a love your neighbor in the verb sense of what we can physically do for them, although praying for them and knowing their needs to support them emotionally is arguably more important.

But getting on a ladder and cleaning your elderly neighbor's gutters or bringing a meal to a family in crisis requires a body. Similarly, although we love God with the immaterial part of us—heart, soul, and mind—we also love and worship Him by using our bodies. We raise our hands in worship, maybe sing and play a musical instrument, or get on our knees before Him. And what we do for a living needs bodies too. We need our bodies to do all kinds of things, but again, what our bodies *look like* in all these activities is irrelevant!

## Overhauled!

Remember Ted with his rusty but trusty muscle car? Then this reality TV program about custom cars comes along, takes Ted's car, and makes it way better than it ever was. They completely disassemble the car down to every nut and bolt and repaint and restore every single little thing. They give it far superior components, like a new, more powerful engine, a killer stereo system, and much better brakes. They remove all the rust, smooth out the dents, and give it an awesome paint job. The result is a car that is, at heart, the original car but is so much better that it's unrecognizable as the same car.

Our physical bodies are headed for the same thing at the resurrection of the righteous. We will "put on" immortality and then have perfect, imperishable bodies. How should that reality change our thinking, and how much should we care what our bodies look like now since that "now" is only a fleeting vapor's breath compared to eternity?

Or we could ask Ted who has a restored, new, custom car what he thinks about all the effort and mental focus he put into what his car previously looked like. "A big waste of time and attention," he might say. "It was never even close to what I wanted." After all, cars are made to take us places, so it hardly matters what they look like while doing it.

## S.O.P.s and Side Effects

No doubt you have seen the commercials on TV for medications that enumerate all kinds of side effects. All those side effects are bad, and most seem worse than actually just living with whatever the medication is supposed to "fix." Let me define what I mean by *side effects*. A side effect is a secondary result of a primary action and may or may not be intended or even wanted. In the case of many medications, the side effect is unavoidable and also unwanted because it is detrimental.

When it comes to taking care of our bodies, there is one side effect that most of us *do* want, and that is to look good! So how is looking the way we want to a side effect? Simply put, it's the result of *how we live*. And the result of how we live is obvious to all. It shows!

Usually, we don't live like we ought to, so we don't look like we want to. But if we are living according to God's will, we will like the side effects it produces. When I say, "how we live," I mean what our daily practices are. Like, how we eat and exercise, how much we sleep, the time we spend in God's word and in prayer, what we do for a job, what our hobbies are, and everything else we do. All of these should be consistent habits.

I call these habits Standard Operating Procedure, or S.O.P.s. If we want to be healthy and fit, it can't be an on-again, off-again effort. We have to just live in such a way that it all results in being healthy. Going "on a diet" to get a certain result or making a big, unusual push to really improve fitness is futile because even if we accomplish what we want, when we go back to our normal daily habits, we also return to our condition before the diet or additional exercise.

I've said to people many, many times, "I don't try to look like this; it's just a result of how I live." My consistent, daily habits result in my being healthy and fit, which in turn has the result or side effect of looking fit, which means looking the way I like. It has to be in that order, or it doesn't work.

So, establish S.O.P.s that produce health and well-being, and over the course of time, you will improve muscle tone, cardiovascular condition, and flexibility, and you will also incrementally lose body fat. This last point is key and really takes the pressure off the desire to lose weight. It *will* happen; we just have to be patient and wait for it. We've got to let it be a side effect and not a main focus.

## That's Not Good for You!

We've heard that phrase from more than just our moms. Probably wives have said it to their husbands, and well-meaning friends have said it to you. After I started to eat really low carb, more than a few people said it wasn't good for me. Well, more than a year later, I am still eating the keto way and have never felt better or been in better physical condition.

It's not just the low carb though. It's that I strive to do only what is good for me, especially with what I eat. My food intake is *only* what is good for me! No compromise. Maybe you wonder what I mean by compromise. For me, compromise is eating something that has a negative effect on my body. Mainly, it is foods that are too high in carbohydrates or foods that contain both high amounts of carbs and fat. No matter how good it might taste, I don't think we have the right to negatively affect our bodies just to get emotional enjoyment from it.

Believe me, I know what it is like to not give a lick about what food is doing to my body, and for years and years, I suffered the consequences. So, I am fairly black and white on this matter. But we all have our convictions before God, so I surely don't expect you to have the same sentiments.

I also take this "only what is good for me" thing into every other area of my life. With exercise, mainly weight training, I constantly pray that I will do "only and all" that is good for me. For my heart and soul and emotional well-being, I seek the same thing. I say, "only and all," because there certainly is a "not enough" and a "too much" in everything. We can even read the Bible too much!

There is a time, a place, and a limit to everything, and being such individuals as we are with such different personalities, I must leave it up to your own personal convictions about what is enough and too much. But I recommend this prayer: "God grant me wisdom to know and the courage and commitment to do only and all that is good for me."

But consider this final thought. We are not our own. We are bought and paid for by Jesus, and we are God's property and stewards of these bodies. Do we not have a responsibility to care for them as well as we possibly can? And if our theology is right, then we believe that God does everything for our good and for His glory. So how can we do any less?

## CHAPTER 12

# What We Look Like

I made the point in the last chapter that what our bodies look like doesn't matter, but how they function does. And it doesn't really matter what the rest of us—clothes, hairstyle, makeup, jewelry—looks like either. This is where I'll finish the statement I made in the last chapter: "It doesn't matter what you look like; it's who you are that matters…." The rest of it goes like this: "But who you are makes you what you look like."

### We Look Like Who We Are

Slow down and picture these kinds of people: bodybuilders, long distance runners, sumo wrestlers, professional bike racers, football linebackers, tennis players, and jockeys in horse racing. Consider a lean, massively muscular bodybuilder and a bulky sumo wrestler. Each may weigh 330 pounds and be healthy and fit, but they sure do look different.

So what's the point? Who we *are* makes us what we look like! Now, admittedly, these examples of what bodies look like are based on particular professions, but people are in these professions because of *who they are*. I mean, jockeys can't be sumo wrestlers. We have to live according to who we are, and who we are makes us what we look like.

Another aspect to these kinds of people is their clothing—how they dress. When they put on a uniform or whatever else they wear for their profession, we can see who they are. Businessmen, postal workers, road construction flagmen, and police officers are also easy to identify, regardless of body condition. Again, we look like who we are.

Aside from professions, we still look like who we are but in the sense of expressing who we are through hairstyle, clothing choices, jewelry, tattoos, and more. We make these choices based on where we grew up, the culture we live in, the family we have or don't have, and just our general experience of life. In a sense, we can hardly help who we are and consequently what we look like.

For example, the Maasai people of Kenya with their colorful red clothing and elaborate jewelry are far different than the much plainer (and furrier) clothing of the Inupiat people of northern Alaska. The choices these two very different people groups make are based on their culture and society, and so they look like who they are. We do the same. But some may say—

## "Who Cares What You Look Like?!"

I think few people can say this and really mean it, except for little Johnny on Sunday morning who has to wear a suit he feels confined in, a tie that feels like it chokes him, uncomfortable shoes that make his feet hurt, and combed hair he isn't allowed to touch until church is over. And probably most kids in general when they are still young enough could not give a rip about what they look like. For them, it's all about what they are *doing,* and they have no concept of why mom complains about grass stains and dirty faces.

We ought to be similar, caring far more about how we're functioning and what we're doing than what we look like doing it. I mean, when little Johnny gets home from church, he's in his jeans, T-shirt inside out, and sneakers on the wrong feet, but he's going!

He's doing! And he doesn't care what he looks like! For us adults, we *do* care what we look like, and we ought to—to some extent—but we are probably far more concerned than we should be.

## Beauty and the Beast

I think what stuff looks like matters to God because we see so much color and variety in His creation. Not every color, texture, or composition of a plant or animal is necessary for its proper functioning. Take horses, for instance. They could all be a boring brown, and that wouldn't change their function at all. But the variety of breeds and their colors are amazing. Or how about guitars? They could all be the same color, and that would not change their function one bit. And what about centipedes? Despite the prefix in the name, which signifies 100, centipedes always have an uneven number of pairs of legs, ranging among different species from 30 to 354. So, they never will have just 100 legs. Who needs all those legs?! Surely they could function as well with a few less? Anyway, the point is that while God made things to function, He also incorporated beauty and complexity into creation.

But there is also ugliness. Now, I know about how beauty is in the eye of the beholder, but the phrase "a face only a mother could love" came from somewhere. Or how about wildebeests or the horrible, ugly, screeching sound that pigs make when you try to restrain them? Ugly! I know it's a defensive mechanism, but poisonous tree frogs use their beautiful, bright, colorful appearance to ward off attack. Certainly God has a purpose for the way things look and for their aesthetic appeal, so I think we should too.

## We Have to Look Like Something....

Recently, I watched a video of a professional bodybuilder wearing a tank top and walking down a public sidewalk. The guy was massively muscular and lean, like the comic book Hulk character, except he wasn't green. It was amazing to see how people responded—taking pictures, standing, and gawking, some pointing from a distance. And the women, well, they had to get their hands on the guy! Of course, that was just to stand next to him to get a picture with him, all because of his body.

Now, I can understand that when you see something visually impressive and above average, you'll want to take a look. That is true for me in regard to the breed of Friesian horses. I think they are the most beautiful, elegant, and soulful looking horse there is, and any time I see one, that horse has my full attention. Then there are all the tattoos I have that are impressive, above average, and eye-catching. I get that people want to take a look, and since these tattoos are all about theology, it can lead to meaningful conversation. As I have been emphasizing, what our bodies look like is irrelevant to how they function, but we at least have to look like *something*. And we do, but probably not how we want to.

It's okay to want to look a certain way as long as our motives are pure, and our first priority is how our body functions. But I will be the first to admit that I *care what my body looks like*! I also care what my car looks like! And also, what my guitars look like. My first priority when I bought my acoustic, bass, and electric guitars was what they looked like. Stupid I know, but that is the truth. Probably being an artist and very appreciative of the visual had a lot to do with it, but my electric guitar, while I love the look of it, is much more suited to heavy metal music. Since I only play on the praise team at church, I have to tone down that beast of a guitar, but it sure looks cool!

So I know what it is like to really care about what stuff looks like, but as I've emphasized, it has to be function over form.

## A Personal Example

In 2012, I had a difficulty with some Christians who thought my appearance was immodest and meant to attract attention. Since they were members of the church I attend, I thought a good solution was to write a paper and explain my appearance to them. What I looked like then is almost what I look like now. I shave my head except for a short Mohawk, I have full-sleeve tattoos on both arms, I wear well-fitting T-shirts that have "Disciple of Jesus Christ" printed on them, and I wear tailored military camouflage pants and tactical boots (and other assorted militant-looking gear). The pants and shirts fit like they do because loose-fitting, baggy-looking clothes seem sloppy and unorganized to me, which equates (in my mind) to a lack of discipline, intentionality, and seriousness. Obviously, this is my personal view and not one I would expect or suggest that anyone else have. But it is currently my reality, so I must live accordingly.

I have included this paper here because it expresses most of what I want to get across in this chapter, although from a more personal perspective with more elaboration. Much of it sounds like stuff I have written in this book so far, so that scores some points for consistency!

## As Concerns My Appearance....

Some would say that my appearance needs an explanation, but frankly, I wish people would just get over it. There are far more important things in this world than what I or anyone else looks like. But since I am writing this paper to explain my appearance, I suppose I must put down some content and get it over with.

### *It Doesn't Matter What You Look Like*

As my daughter was growing up, it became apparent that she was going to be somewhat short as an adult. I began to emphasize that it didn't matter what she looked like but that who she was as a person was what was important. I frequently used the phrase, "You may be short on the outside, but you're tall on the inside." Now an adult, she is indeed "tall on the inside," and her short stature is of little consequence to her. When she was about 12 years old, she wanted to dye her hair purple. I said to her, "That's fine. It doesn't matter what you look like. It's who you are that matters." I emphasized that in every way I could as she grew up.

When I say it doesn't matter what you look like, I do not mean you should have no care or concern for your appearance. Certainly, we should make ourselves presentable and be clean and neat, and wear clothes that are appropriate to who we are. When I emphasized to my daughter that it was who she was as a person that was most important, I knew that having her focus on that and placing her value in that rather than her appearance would naturally cause her to dress in a way that was congruent with her personality and character. So it has turned out to be.

## Look Like Who You Are

Of course, we all dress according to our personality and character. I don't know anyone who dresses in a way that is contrary to what they like or what they are comfortable with. I am no different in that regard. The way I dress expresses who I am. It's what I like, and I am very comfortable with that. To dress in a different style would be uncomfortable for me, as it indeed would be for anyone.

For example, let's say someone in sandals and shorts begins attending a legalistic type of church. Almost all the other men wear suits. The leaders determine that the visitor's appearance shows that he is irreverent, and they ask him to begin wearing a suit. The visitor would be uncomfortable in a suit because it is not his style. It would also be hypocritical because it would project an image of him that is false. He looks like who he is, and his appearance does not determine whether he is reverent or irreverent.

## *You Look Like Something to Everyone*

Everything about us communicates something to people. Surely misconceptions abound when a person is assessed only by their appearance. I think there are as many interpretations of what you look like as there are people who are doing the looking. I had a person, a stranger I had gotten into a conversation with, say to me, "You're not what I expected." When I questioned them, they intimated that they hadn't expected me to be so kind, knowledgeable, and intelligent.

Since we look like something to everyone and everyone looks on the outward appearance, I believe our outward appearance should reflect, as much as is possible, what is in our heart. That way, when a person looks at our outward appearance, they can better know who we are. I mean, look at anyone who wears a T-shirt with some kind of logo or something written on it, and you'll immediately know what they like or believe in. Obviously, you can't tell with people who have nothing on their shirts, but their choice of clothing can communicate something about them. You may see a middle-aged man wearing khaki pants and a similarly colored polo shirt and brown loafers and assume he is boring and uninspiring. You could be right or wrong, but there is no telling until you actually talk to him. But based on his appearance, you would probably not have looked twice at him, and so any opportunity for conversation would have passed by unnoticed.

## *No One Is an Original*

When it comes to it, the clothes we wear are just variations of what everyone else is wearing. We take this shirt and those pants and pick those shoes and put it together, and then we think we're unique. We're not. We just put our outfit together a little differently than the next guy, but it's really all the same stuff. Surely, you've seen someone wearing camouflage army pants or someone with a T-shirt that has a Christian message on it, and another person who has on footwear similar to mine, and yet a fourth person who carries their belongings in a fanny pack. I'm not much different. I just put all this together in one outfit.

People choose what they wear for their own reasons (some are hard to fathom), and I am no different, although I think I am much more intentional than most. The reason I put my clothes together the way I do is because my heart tells me I am a disciplined, devoted, and passionate soldier of Jesus Christ. I am in a war, and a battle rages within me every day to fight evil. My heart, soul, and mind are the theater where forces beyond my comprehension take up arms and engage in conflict.

The massive power and will of Satan pours temptation into me with the blasphemous and ungodly intent to cause me to transgress against the ordained will of God. That is pitted against the infinite dominion and sovereignty of God, who is at work within me annihilating my sin and even slaughtering temptation before it can become sin. It is beyond finding out how something of such magnitude can occur within me.

What kind of strength must God exert in me to enable me to endure it? It must be staggering. But He not only enables me to endure but grants that I may conquer, and not only that I may conquer but to be more than a conqueror by turning the vanquished foe into a servant that benefits the cause of good. It is a hard war, but it is a good war and one I am as committed as I can be to fight.

## *A Wartime Lifestyle*

A popular Christian pastor and author talks about this war and suggests that we should have a "wartime lifestyle" mindset. His main tenet is that we must live our lives as simply as possible to advance the cause of Christ and be committed to winning the battle every moment. We must not let our vigilance be disrupted by discomfort or indulge in things that aren't essential to the war effort.

I certainly am oriented to see all of life as a war. The spiritual battle is real and must be fought every moment of every day. I get that. I really get that, and I love the fight, and I love the victory. I am all about ordering my life and maximizing every aspect of it to serve God's cause in this world. I want to leave no stone unturned in this quest, and I don't want to be weighed down with anything that is unnecessary to achieve victory. That is the mindset of a soldier. It is my mindset, and consequently I express it in my appearance.

In addition, I believe that the goal of a Christian woman's life is not to make expression of the self ( body or character) the main thing, but to express God and His all-satisfying greatness, to promote His cause and proclaim His truth. Excessive preoccupation with what we look like is a sign that self, not God, has moved to the center.

## *We All Attract Attention*

People look at other people. People are attracted to other people. People notice other people. There are numerous reasons for that, whether it be that a person is a huge bodybuilder; dressed in dirty, raggedy clothes; wearing one of those gaudy Christmas sweaters; have on pajamas and fuzzy boots at the mall; dress in an expensive suit with alligator shoes; or whatever. You can't help that people will look at you, but for whatever reason, they will look, maybe not all the time or in every circumstance, but we all get looked at. Or even if someone is walking down the road, you look when you drive by.

Certainly, it comes down to what is in your heart and your motives for how you appear. For instance, does a Marine put on his uniform in order to attract the attention and admiration of people? Hardly! It's just what he wears because that's who he is.

## *We All Want Attention*

People want attention because they need to be heard and understood, whether it's in a marriage, in a friendship, at a job with your boss, ordering fast food, or trying to sell newspapers. Remember the newspaper boys that used to stand on the street corner yelling, "Extra, extra, read all about it"? Now, they were definitely trying to attract attention but with the intent that people would buy a paper and read the news. It is necessary that the newspaper boy attract attention so he can get the news out, but he isn't about getting attention for himself.

I do not want to attract attention to myself for my own sake, but I do want to draw people's attention to me so I can get the good news into their hands.

*A Little History*

Years ago, I used to wear "normal" clothes and have "normal" hair. Going farther back, I used to be 55 pounds overweight and wore clothes that I hoped would hide me from all onlookers. My heart was not for God but was all about what I looked like because I felt ugly. Being obsessed with my bad appearance, I didn't want to be looked at. My appearance communicated who I was, and since I was overweight and didn't keep myself very well, I hated what it communicated. Back then, it was all about what people thought of me based on what I looked like. It made for a terrible experience of life.

More than 20 years ago, I lost 55 pounds to come down to a normal weight. In that process, with my identity still wrapped up in how I looked, I began to seek attention—and I got it, mostly from men at the gym. But it was still a terrible experience of life because it was still all about me and how I looked.

As I started going back to church, I saw a new audience, a Christian audience, and began dressing up to be seen. I had never worn dresses in my life before, but I recognized the church setting as a place I could put on dresses and suits and look really good. I also altered my behavior to come off as a disciplined, godly woman. I got lots of compliments for both my supposed character and how I looked. I have looked back so many times at where my focus was and what I valued, and I can only see what a waste of life it was.

As I matured in Christ, God gradually showed me how vain I was and changed my heart and focus to seek all my joy and satisfaction in Him. One obvious change is that I stopped dressing up for Sunday morning. I had resisted for a long time the conviction that I was a distraction or even a temptation to some of my brothers in Christ. I quite enjoyed getting looked at up and down, and also the looks that lasted longer than they should.

It's just sickening to look back on that. I wish someone had told me back then to tone it down or had raised the issue of pride and the sin of wanting to draw attention to myself so I could be admired. It's ironic that now, when all my heart is to point people to Christ, I get called out for wanting attention for myself or that pride is an issue or whatever.

## *Getting Personal . . . and Specific*

Now I want to address certain points of my appearance and describe why and what and how. I mean, I didn't just wake up one day and say, "I think I'll shave my head and start wearing military clothing!"

It has been a long process and one in which God has gradually scraped off the façade of who I wanted people to think I was into just plain "being who I am." I make no apologies and only offer explanations when I am asked. I remember one of my church friends—one among many who have the same sentiment—commenting that she wished she could be as free as I am from the tyranny of what people think of her. I replied, "Well, there'd be a lot of us who would look significantly different, I'm sure. For instance, you wouldn't have to color your hair anymore." She smiled, put her hand to her hair, and said, "But I'd be all gray!"

I am an artist and therefore very visual in my orientation to reality. Truth becomes pictures to me. It's similar to when the pastor put things in the bulletin to remind us of his message. I still have the broken piece of pottery he gave everyone to remind us to be humble in regard to the story about a retarded kid named Billy who got picked on at summer camp. He once gave us stones that we were to confer our sin on and then cast into a lake. He gave us playing cards to remind us to respond properly to the hand God had dealt us, and a Lego block to ask us, "What are you building with your life?"

My clothing and appearance are full of these visual cues for me. That is especially true for my tattoos. I have them primarily for my own benefit. Their meaning is not readily apparent to anyone else and can only be understood if I explain what they mean. For example, I will soon have the international symbol for "biohazard" tattooed near my elbow. Its meaning is primarily for me, but I am happy to explain it to anyone who asks. Secondarily, my tattoos are there, if God should so choose, to use them as a conversation starter to lead people to Christ.

My militaristic style of dress is a huge visual cue to me and makes me feel more serious, disciplined, and committed to "walk in a manner worthy of the gospel." The type of pants I wear are called BDUs, which is short for "battle dress uniform." When I get dressed, it signifies to me that I am preparing for battle and taking this life and calling of God very seriously, to live it as professionally and successfully as I can.

Soldiers have a very high degree of self-discipline, integrity, loyalty, and deadly commitment to the cause. They are militant, and my dressing in a similar manner to a soldier cultivates and encourages these qualities in me. It also fosters a state of mind that better enables me to respond appropriately to whatever circumstance I may be in. Another motive for how I dress is that I want to express visually that I am a "good soldier of Jesus Christ" (2 Tim. 2:3–4), not only to myself, but to others as well. I want people to immediately know who I am and what I believe. That's why my clothes are labeled with "Disciple of Jesus Christ." That has led to countless instances of speaking about the truth of God to others.

My hairstyle expresses the radical and militant extremism that the Christian faith requires us to have if we are to be fruitful and successful. Again, my hairstyle is more about what it says to me than what other people may think.

I wear a chain necklace with a cross on it to signify to myself that I am "bearing my own cross." Every day, before I put it on, I kneel down on one knee before God as my King and proclaim to Him that I am willingly taking up my cross to bear it at whatever cost to me, and I ask God to fill me with the strength and grace to be able to do so. At the same time, I offer myself as a living sacrifice and an instrument of righteousness to be used by God in whatever way He decrees. At the end of the day, I am on my knees before Him, admitting that I failed to bear my cross as He commanded and asking to be made more able to bear it the next day.

I have a piercing just below my lip that reminds me to "Let no unwholesome word proceed from your mouth, but only such *a word* as is good for edification according to the need of *the moment*, so that it will give grace to those who hear" (Eph. 4:29). One of my earrings signifies to me that I am committed to Christ as a lifelong slave (Exod. 21:6).

## Superheroes and the Human Physique

Another aspect of my appearance is my physical condition. I take it as seriously as my spiritual condition and seek to be as fit as I believe God has called me to be. I am a steward of this body, and it is my duty to be as healthy and well as I can be. A nice benefit of being healthy and fit is that it produces an appearance that is a benefit to me.

I have a very high regard for the beauty and symmetry of the human form. Superheroes such as the Hulk and Batman, and athletes such as bodybuilders exemplify and exaggerate the human form in a very powerful and appealing way. To me, their powerful and fit appearance represents emotional and spiritual strength, as well as being an image of victory. I draw a lot of inspiration from superheroes and bodybuilders and have many images and action figures of them in my drawing room.

I wish I could look like a superhero, partly because I sometimes feel like one but also because I don't really look that much better than average. Still, my physical appearance as I am serves as a visual cue and is motivating in the same way my military style of dress is.

## *A Word about Spirituality*

Since we're talking about appearance, I have said little about my attention to the spiritual aspect or my inner being. That is far more important to me than what I look like, and I am even more intentional about doing all I can to maximize my growth in Christlikeness. As much effort as I make to look the way I do physically and with the clothes I wear, I am far more concerned that I look like Jesus in a spiritual sense and in the way I relate to others. I am more than willing to admit how blind, deaf, pitiful, and wretchedly far I am from being like Jesus.

## *Putting It All Together*

If you take all of what I've explained and described about my clothes, tattoos, hairstyle, jewelry, and physical condition and combine it all, what I am is a person who is doing all I can to maximize and optimize every aspect of my being in order to be as fit as I can to glorify God and advance His Kingdom.

Finally, I want to state emphatically that everything I've described about the way I look and how I dress is not necessary for me to live a passionate and obedient life. But it is what I prefer and how I feel comfortable. It is just plain what I like. It's who I am. All the visual cues provided by my clothing, hairstyle, tattoos, and physical condition are very motivating and of great benefit in encouraging me and reminding me of who I am and what my mission is in this world.

CHAPTER 13

# Why We Live

So how does a person finish a book like this? Seems like I've said all that needs saying, but it's not sitting well with me that the book should end on the previous chapter that was all about us and what we look like. It's not about us; it's about *God*. It's about what our purpose is in this life, why we are alive, and what God has saved us to do. And it doesn't really matter what we look like while we're doing it.

## Mission: Impossible

"Your mission, should you choose to accept it. . . ." In that old TV show and the more recent movies, the secret agent guy and his team never listened to the tape and then said, "Well, forget that, let's go to the beach instead!" They always accepted the mission, knowing that the fate of many people's lives depended on it. And to be accurate, the mission was never impossible. They always got it done, so I don't know why that was the title. Maybe it was to build drama.

Anyway, we are in a similar situation, but our mission is *real*, also not optional, and indeed quite possible. We are commanded to "Go therefore and make disciples of all the nations" (Matt. 28:19). That's our mission. Whatever else we do in our lives is just the means by which our mission is supported and enabled.

## Why Are We Alive?

A popular Christian apologist said that the two greatest days in our lives are the day we were born and the day we find out why. "What is the meaning of life?" is a question that has been asked by far more people than have ever come up with an accurate answer. As believers in Jesus, we know that the meaning of life is God Himself. He created us to worship Him so He would be glorified. When we worship God, we behold Him, we see Him, and we experience Him, and thus rejoice in how good and glorious He is, which fills us with joy and satisfaction. This is what every human being desires. But without knowing God, people futilely seek satisfaction in everything but God.

Likely, we have done the same thing ourselves, so we know the pain, disappointment, and hopelessness of trying to satisfy ourselves with the things of this world. But now, since we know the truth and have been reconciled to God, He has given us the mission of telling the truth to those who don't know it. It's as simple as that. It's why you and I are alive. And speaking of being alive, consider this:

> *I have been crucified with Christ; and it is no longer I who live, but Christ lives in me; and the* life *which I now live in the flesh I live by faith in the Son of God, who loved me and gave Himself up for me.*
> —Galatians 2:20

We are alive, and yet Paul says we are *not alive,* but *Christ* lives in us. It is His presence in us that gives us true life—spiritual life. Without that, we would be as the rest of the world, separated from God and dead in sin and transgressions. But we are *alive* and duty-bound to proclaim the truth of the gospel to the world so they will know why *they* are alive.

I wrote a short story many, many years ago that makes this point, and so it seems a good place to share it with you.

## The Story of Mr. Pencil

"I just don't how I got to be where I am," began Mr. Pencil.

But Mr. Paper interrupted, "Never mind that. Do you know *why* you're here? I've been wondering for a long time why *I'm* here, and I haven't figured it out."

Mr. Pencil looked puzzled as he looked thoughtfully at Mr. Paper.

"The thing is," continued Mr. Paper, "it seems like I've been waiting my whole life for something, and I don't know what it is." He looked down at the ground with a vacant, sad kind of look.

Mr. Pencil felt a stab of compassion and said, "I wish I could help...."

Tears welled up in Mr. Paper and he cried out, "I've never once felt satisfied or useful to anyone!"

Mr. Pencil moved closer to comfort him but didn't know what to say.

"I mean, I feel so—so horribly *blank*." By now, Mr. Paper was all wilted over in a hopeless kind of gloom.

Mr. Pencil was searching for something to say when a thought struck him. "Say, I used to know someone else named Mr. Paper, but he looked a lot different than you."

Mr. Paper looked up expectantly, sniffled, and said, "Different how?"

But suddenly Mr. Pencil said, "Look! Someone's coming."

Mr. Paper looked in the direction Mr. Pencil was gesturing. Mr. Paper looked intently for a moment and said in a hushed tone, "Look at him. What's the matter with him?"

Mr. Pencil answered, "I don't know. He looks really funny."

By now the stranger was near enough, so that Mr. Paper and Mr. Pencil prepared to greet him. He bounced up and stopped in front of them. He was only about one-fourth as tall as Mr. Pencil, rectangular, pink, and smudged with black.

"Hi! I'm Mr. Eraser!" he bubbled. "How you guys doing?"

"Well," started Mr. Pencil, but he was startled when Mr. Paper blurted out, "What's the *matter* with you?"

"Matter? Nothing's the matter," said Mr. Eraser. "I'm as happy as I can be!"

"But you're all dirty looking, and it looks like the top of you is worn off," said Mr. Pencil

Eraser looked up briefly as if to try to see the top of himself and then said exuberantly, "Well, silly, I've been doing my job. Nothing makes me happier than that!"

Mr. Paper looked at Mr. Pencil in a puzzled way, and he returned the look.

"What do you mean . . . *job*?" questioned Mr. Paper, feeling a sense of expectation.

But instead of answering, Eraser bounced back from them a bit and looked each of them up and down and said, "You know, you should talk about someone looking funny. Look at you two."

They looked down at themselves and then at each other and then back to Mr. Eraser.

"Well, what do you mean?" said Mr. Paper, suddenly feeling naked.

"Well, look at you, there's not a mark on you. You're *blank*!" said Mr. Eraser.

The word *blank* hit Mr. Paper like a physical blow, and he crumpled to the ground, bursting into tears. "I *know* I'm blank! Why is it so depressing?!" he trailed off, sobbing.

Eraser bounced up next to him and said, "Hey, it'll be all right, once you know what you were made for."

Mr. Paper's sobbing lessened, and he took a few deep breaths. Then he said weakly and with a note of hope, "Yeah?"

"Sure!" exclaimed Eraser. "Once you know what you were made for, you're on your way to being truly happy!"

Mr. Pencil suddenly interjected, "Say, wait a minute. I know plenty of guys named Paper who are perfectly happy, and they all look like him—blank." Mr. Paper winced at the sound of the word, but Mr. Pencil continued, "Are you saying that Paper can't be happy being blank?"

"Yeah, just like you can't be happy without having a usable point."

Mr. Pencil felt a twinge of defensiveness and said, "What do you mean, a *point*?"

"Well, pencils can't do what they were made to do without a point," answered Eraser.

Mr. Pencil was unsatisfied with Eraser's answer and said, "But what *is* a point? All the pencils I've ever seen look just like me."

A thought occurred to Eraser, and he said, "Say, you ought to come and meet Mr. H. B. Pencil. I've just been working with him over there, and you, Mr. Paper, ought to meet this Frenchman I know named Mr. Papier. Come on!" Eraser bounced off, followed closely by Mr. Paper and Mr. Pencil who were quite interested in meeting Eraser's acquaintances.

After a few minutes, they rounded a corner and suddenly heard, "Hey, Eraser! There you are! Come on over. We need you." But before Mr. Paper or Mr. Pencil could focus on who was speaking, Eraser suddenly rose way up in the air and came down on someone who they presumed to be Mr. Papier and began scrubbing back and forth. The moment this happened, Mr. Paper let out a shriek of terror and ducked, as if expecting a blow, and Mr. Pencil stiffened as he felt a wave of fear.

"What . . . wh . . . what the . . . what happened?" sputtered Mr. Paper.

Eraser gleefully called out, "It's Almighty Artist using me. You can't see him because he's invisible."

Mr. Paper became very anxious and worried, and he backed up a bit. Eraser stopped erasing and suddenly rose up and came straight at them. Mr. Pencil jumped behind Mr. Paper, who fell flat on his face, quivering in fear. But Mr. Eraser landed right in front of them and said, "Hey, you guys, don't worry."

Mr. Pencil moved away from Mr. Paper and said, "*I'm* not worried, and I didn't think your trick of flying through the air was very funny either." He seemed quite put off and turned to look off into the distance, but his attention was sharply grabbed by Mr. H. B. Pencil. He was gliding around on Mr. Papier at a 45-degree angle. Mr. Pencil was awestruck. Being a pencil himself, he couldn't fathom how Mr. H. B. could do that.

Mr. Pencil rushed over and cried out, "Hey! How . . . stop it! How can you *do* that?" But he suddenly saw the bottom of H. B. and grimaced horribly, and said, "Ugh! Look at you! You look . . . horrible!"

"What?" said H. B. innocently. He looked down at himself and said, "Oh, that's my point! You don't have one I see."

"No, and I never want one either. Ick!" Mr. Pencil retorted. His attention was caught by Mr. Papier who had stood up. Mr. Pencil burst out, "Oh, and you! You look *awful*! What *is* that on you?"

"What?" said Mr. Papier looking at himself as best he could.

"It's the artwork of Almighty Artist," said H. B. "And I think it's beautiful."

Mr. Papier beamed at H. B. and said, "Well, thanks. I rather agree, *bon ami*."

A thin, little voice came from behind Mr. Pencil, startling him. "What is it like?"

Mr. Paper moved past Mr. Pencil and right up to Mr. Papier, who answered, "What's *what* like?"

Mr. Paper was kind of dreamy and elaborated, "What's it like, not being . . . being . . . uh. . . ."

He felt pained, and before he could finish, Mr. Pencil yelled out harshly, "*Blank*! He wants to know what it feels like to not be *blank*! Ha!"

Mr. Paper quivered under the blow but stood up straighter and ignored Mr. Pencil.

Eraser shot a look at Pencil that would have splintered him to pieces if it could. Eraser moved closer to Mr. Paper in a supportive, kind way, and Mr. Papier glared steadily at Mr. Pencil as he said, "I don't *ever* use the 'B' word because I know how much it hurts when you don't know Almighty Artist."

Mr. Pencil just stood and glared back, quite pleased with himself for having had such an effect on everyone.

Mr. Paper was beginning to feel hope and said, "Please, Mr. Papier, who is Almighty Artist? Can he help me to not feel so . . . so bad?"

Eraser spoke and Mr. Paper turned to him, "Are you willing to begin doing what you were made to do?"

Mr. Paper was thinking about an answer when Mr. Pencil interrupted. "You fool! Don't you know that you'll have to look hideous like that *chose affreuse*?"

Mr. Paper spun around and fairly yelled, "You're the fool! You don't even know what you're talking about! Mr. Papier is a work of *art*! Can't you *see*? Don't you *feel* it? This is what we've both been waiting for our whole lives! Don't you see that there is something bigger than ourselves? This is what we were *made* for!"

Mr. Pencil became angrier and yelled back, "Yah! What do *you* know, Mr. Blankety Blank! I don't buy *any* of it! There is no such thing as Almighty *anything*!" Mr. Pencil took a big breath to continue his tirade, but his words turned quickly to screams of panic and terror as he was suddenly lifted high into the air. His horrific shrieks faded quickly from hearing as he disappeared like a shot over the horizon.

Mr. Paper stood there speechless and staring. When he finally looked back at Eraser, H.B. and Mr. Papier looked very grave. "What happened to Mr. Pencil?" Mr. Paper asked tentatively. He had a foreboding that it wasn't good.

The three looked back and forth at each other, wondering who would answer because none of them really wanted to describe what they knew had happened. Finally, it seemed to fall on Eraser who said somewhat slowly, "Sooner or later, that's what happens to everyone who refuses to do what they were made to do."

Mr. Paper asked anxiously, "Well, *what* happened?"

Mr. Papier shivered and could only manage to whisper, "Fire."

"You . . . you mean . . . burned up?" stuttered Mr. Paper, feeling more frightened than he ever had in his life. He looked quickly back and forth at each of them.

When H. B. took a breath to speak, Mr. Paper looked square at him and waited breathlessly. H. B. paused and looked in a pained way at each of his friends and then back to Mr. Paper. "Well," he started slowly, "not exactly *burned* up, but *burning* up."

"For how long?" asked Mr. Paper.

"For*ever*," said Mr. Eraser.

Mr. Paper turned to him, incredulous, and said, "But how can that be? I've . . . I've seen *ashes*, you know. I mean, doesn't it ever get over?"

Mr. Eraser just shook his head slowly, and H. B. said, "That's just how it is . . . there."

Mr. Paper stared for a second, and then tears started streaming down him and he fell down flat, terrified of his own fate.

They all rushed to gather around him, and Eraser said excitedly, "No, no, Mr. Paper, don't be scared. Almighty Artist *loves* you. He *made* you."

"But what about Mr. Pencil? Did Almighty Artist love *him*?"

"Yes, but sadly, Mr. Pencil didn't want to do what Almighty Artist made him for."

Mr. Paper sat up and brightened a bit, "Well, I want to do what I was made for!" They were all filled with joy, but suddenly a frown came upon Mr. Paper, and all paused in their reveling. "Will I be safe from . . . from being burned?" said Paper anxiously. "I mean, what if I stop wanting to do what I was made for?"

"Oh well," said Mr. Eraser, "you'll always *want* to be used by Almighty Artist. But maybe you won't always be willing, but He forgives you for that."

"Yeah, besides," interjected H. B., "He makes you different after you accept His purposes for you. Look at Mr. Papier. See how he's not all glossy anymore but kind of dull and just perfect for drawing on? And I never had a point before I knew Almighty Artist, and Eraser's compound was kind of hard and didn't erase at all until Almighty Artist changed him."

"Well, I'm . . . I'm ready to be changed!" proclaimed Mr. Paper.

*I pray that we all would wholly submit ourselves to our Almighty God, that we would be obedient and seek to be holy, and so find in Him all our happiness and joy. May we acknowledge that Jesus died to give us life, that He paid dearly for us, and that we are not our own but belong to Him. May we love God more than anything and as His stewards take the best care of our souls and bodies that we can so we will be as effective as possible in His service. May we be true to who we really are in what we look like and how we live our lives, and boldly proclaim the gospel, speaking the truth in love.*

# About the Author

Charlene Ralph is a born-again Christian, artist, and author with a talent for drawing and writing. Her greatest passion is Jesus Christ—to love Him, know Him, obey Him, proclaim Him, and be more like Him. "He is the driving force in my life and the heartbeat of all I do," she proclaims. Raised in Rochester, New York, in a Christian home with an older brother and twin sister, Char was married at 23, moved west to a small town, and gave birth to her daughter at the age of 26. She serves in the band at her church, Journey Christian, playing bass, lead electric, or acoustic rhythm guitar.

www.ingramcontent.com/pod-product-compliance
Ingram Content Group UK Ltd.
Pitfield, Milton Keynes, MK11 3LW, UK
UKHW031838100225
454898UK00011B/553